MW01633889

LINCOLN ROOM

**UNIVERSITY OF ILLINOIS
LIBRARY**

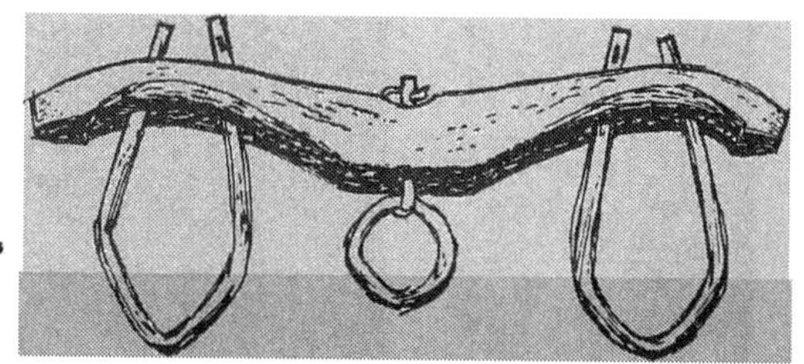

MEMORIAL

the Class of 1901

founded by
HARLAN HOYT HORNER
and
HENRIETTA CALHOUN HORNER

THE RIVALRY

by Norman Corwin

ACTING EDITION

DRAMATISTS
PLAY SERVICE
INC.

DRAMATISTS PLAY SERVICE, INC.

Established by members of the Dramatists' Guild of the Authors' League of America for the handling of the nonprofessional acting rights of members' plays and the encouragement of the nonprofessional theater.

INTIMATE PORTRAITS
By Barrett H. Clark

**MAXIM GORKY — SIDNEY HOWARD
JOHN GALSWORTHY — GEORGE MOORE
EDWARD SHELDON, etc.**

The last book by the author of *Eugene O'Neill, the Man and His Plays, European Theories of the Drama*, etc., is a first-hand informal record of personal friendships, associations and collaborations covering several years and describing with utter frankness a number of well-known playwrights and others whose ideas and off-the-record idiosyncrasies and talk seemed worth preserving. *Intimate Portraits* is in no sense a textbook; it is an uninhibited and rambling series of vivid pictures of men who in their respective fields have helped make contemporary literary and dramatic history.

Cloth bound volume, $2.50

Press Comments:

THE BOOKLIST, American Library Association: *"The subjects live for the reader."*

THE BOOK EXCHANGE, London: *"Especially delightful account . . . written in an easy conversational manner and with complete frankness."*

GEORGE FREEDLEY: *"A wise and knowing book. Mr. Clark doesn't provide you with bright . . . anecdotes that readily can be quoted in a review. His writing and appraisal of his subjects are much too deep and subtle for that. If you want really to know how fine a writer he is and how well he has achieved his aim . . . you'll just have to read* Intimate Portraits *for yourself."*

TALBOT PEARSON (In Dramatics): *"Most delightful volume . . . There is deep affection throughout. Read this book even if you have to buy it."*

ROBERT COLEMAN (N. Y. Mirror): *"Highly illuminating account . . . We were deeply moved . . . Firsthand, exciting material."*

14 EAST 38th STREET, NEW YORK 16, N. Y., U. S. A.

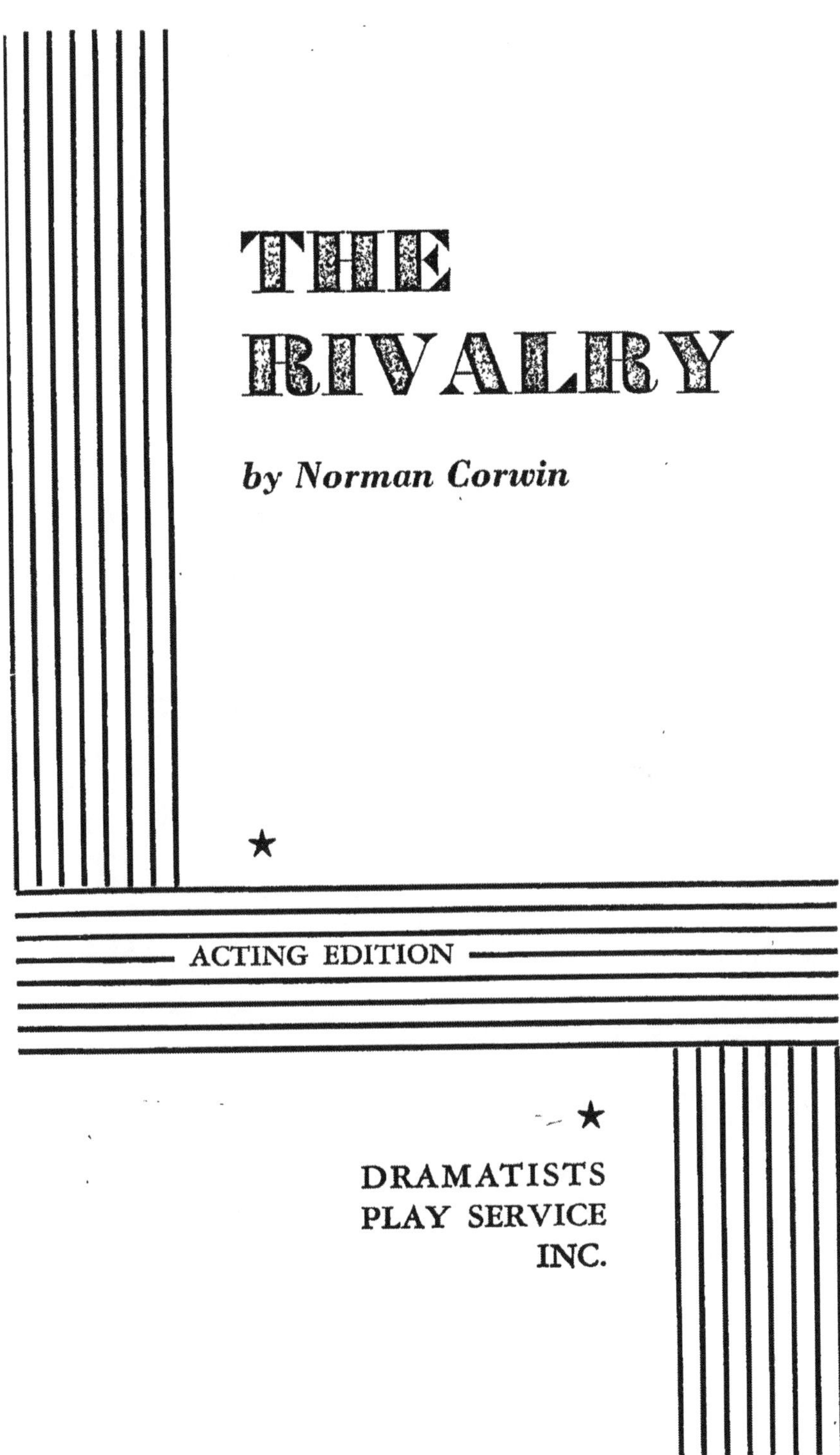

THE RIVALRY

by Norman Corwin

ACTING EDITION

DRAMATISTS
PLAY SERVICE
INC.

For Tony and Diane

The first New York City performance of THE RIVALRY
was presented by Cheryl Crawford and Joel Schenker at the
Bijou Theatre on February 7, 1959. The production was
directed by Mr. Corwin, and the settings were designed by
David Hays. The cast was as follows:

ADELE DOUGLAS .... Nancy Kelly
STEPHEN A. DOUGLAS .... Martin Gabel
ABRAHAM LINCOLN .... Richard Boone

TOWNSPEOPLE

Woodrow Parfrey (Republican Committeeman)
Ailsa Dawson (Lady Democrat)
Jim Campbell

The action takes place in Washington, D. C., and various
cities and towns of Illinois, starting in the summer of 1858.

NOTE: The text of the debates derives from the stenographic record,
although not always used here in their original sequence.

ACT ONE

In the center of a slightly raked plank stage, stands a speaker's platform with removable railings. It suggests the elevated, improvised platforms used at outdoor political rallies in the days long before Madison Square Garden and TV.

The edges of the raked stage go off L and R at an angle divergent from each other, so as to carry the eye into the drapes or shadow at the sides, leaving for the central area whatever is real and immediate, and commending the rest to the infinity of history, out of which our action comes and into which it returns.

The back wall of the stage is susceptible of many treatments, depending on local resources of production. But in any case its needs are little: it must be simple and plain. In the first touring company of THE RIVALRY, *the background consisted of only an American flag of 1858, spread flat. In New York, the back wall was more formidable, consisting of a horizontal red drape crossing the length of the stage (to mask pipes and cross-overs, as well as look pretty); and, rising in front of it, a wide, high blue scrim that reached up out of sight. This formed an inverted T; the area not covered by scrim was the plain brick wall of the house, and it was perfectly at home in the setting.*

On the speaking platform itself are a small table, flanked by two chairs. At the rear of the platform, in the R corner, is a third chair, which will be occupied later by ADELE DOUGLAS.

The lighting scheme throughout is one in which the active element always takes a high key while the others are lower.

If a curtain is not used, the stage should be discovered by the entering audience, lighted with subtle color that suggests neither day nor night—a lighting cue never used during the play itself. The house lights in this case come down, but the stage light remains. After a moment, this lighting too begins to fade, and when it is about half way down, music begins off-stage . . . after which the stage goes to blackness.

As the music diminishes to a muffled tympani, a dim light comes up revealing ADELE *standing at the farthest upstage L corner. She is an impressive figure of a woman, very beautiful, and of whom the descriptive fragments soon to emerge in the first scene, were actually written and said by her contemporaries.*

She comes forward slowly and pauses before she addresses the audience:

ADELE

It is simple now to say it was the greatest debate in history, but greatness is something you have to stand back to see. We were too close at the time; few of us had any idea of the immensity of the tragedy that lay ahead; we did not foresee the fierce outcome of the issues upon which my husband and Mr. Lincoln argued. At first I was reluctant to go along. What woman wants to see her husband in a public mangle? The debates had not even begun, before backs were up. . . . (DOUGLAS *enters L with fire in his eyes, bearing news*)

DOUGLAS

Blast his leathery hide! Damn the arrogance of that man! Adele: do you know that he has the cheek to quibble because I open and close four times to his three? *Somebody* has to open four times in seven debates. My God, you'd think I had pestered HIM for a chance to debate—that he was consenting to something I asked for!

ADELE

How did he quibble?

DOUGLAS

You know the letter I sent him the other day stipulating the times and places of the meetings?

ADELE

Only too well . . . up and down, back and forth, across the
State.

DOUGLAS

Now listen to this: "Although by the terms you propose, you
take four openings to my three, I accede, and thus close the
arrangement. Your obedient servant. . . ." He *accedes!* Damned
decent of him!

ADELE

It doesn't matter who starts the debates—what worries me is
where you'll finish.

DOUGLAS

I will finish, Madam, with the senatorship of Illinois still in
my possession. You are going to see the progressive demolition
of that man. He has asked for it. Moreover, the whole country
will be witness to every detail, what with a swarm of reporters
coming out from the East. Every time my nose is blown, it will
be telegraphed to the country.

ADELE

And every time your nose is tweaked, that will be telegraphed
too.

DOUGLAS

You will never see that happen.

ADELE

How right you are. I will never see it happen because I won't
be there. (STEPHEN *smiles knowingly and starts to remove a
letter from his vest. As he does:*)

DOUGLAS

That again.

ADELE

Not again. Still.

DOUGLAS

(*Has found something in the letter*) Adele, I think I may have found the key to your resistance.

ADELE

It wouldn't be the first time.

DOUGLAS

Do you have the stoicism to hear what people think of you?

ADELE

It depends on what people.

DOUGLAS

Well, Dick Merrick for one.

ADELE

Oh, I'm not afraid of what *he* might say.

DOUGLAS

Listen to this: (*Reading from the letter*) "We won't hear of Adele not coming with you. She will exert a quiet, dignified influence in your behalf, simply by her presence, by the encouragement that presence will give to your friends, and by the restraint she will put upon your enemies—also the enthusiasm she will arouse in those who have the feeling to appreciate so sweet a smile as she can't help smiling. . . ." *Now* will you come?

ADELE

Do you seriously believe all those things about me?

DOUGLAS

(*Embracing her*) You have more constituents than I have, and you know it. Everybody says you're the most beautiful and most accomplished girl in Washington.

ADELE

Vain man, to repeat that to me. —Tell it to me again.

DOUGLAS

They're also saying you've made our home the social White House.

ADELE

If I couldn't manage a better party than your dreary Mr. President Buchanan, I'd return to the nunnery.

DOUGLAS

Now then: are you coming to the debates with me?

ADELE

No, dear, I am not.

DOUGLAS

Adele, let me remind you of something: do you remember that reception at Belleville? (*She nods*) Remember the editor of the German newspaper whose accent fascinated you? And who was so strong for Lincoln?

ADELE

He was also strong for beer.

DOUGLAS

But mainly for *you*, my dear; he was so smitten that he actually changed his party; he's supporting me for re-election. —I swear it's true; he said so himself.

ADELE

Well, I guess I'll just have to face the fact that I'm irresistible.

DOUGLAS

Good; now we're getting somewhere! —Are you coming along with me?

9

ADELE

No!

DOUGLAS

Why?

ADELE

I was against your accepting Lincoln's challenge from the start, and I'm no more receptive to the idea now that you're ready to meet him. (DOUGLAS, *with an amiable gesture of impatience, starts to walk away*) Stephen dear: right now you're more famous than any other public man in America. It's going to be an extraordinary advantage to an ambitious local politician like Lincoln to share the attention that follows you around, and to share it on equal terms. He has everything to gain and nothing to lose.

DOUGLAS

(*Turning and starting back*) I'm from Vermont. . . . I don't run from a challenge! Particularly not on the slavery issue.

ADELE

I'm not asking you to run from a challenge. But the slavery issue is hot enough without your deliberately jumping into the fire. You told me yourself what happened just three years ago —how they burned your effigy right here in Illinois—about those women in Ohio who presented you with thirty pieces of silver—

DOUGLAS

(*Dismissing it*) Oh, they were in an uproar because I jammed through the Nebraska Bill. They've calmed down since—they realize now that all I fought for—and won—was the right of people to VOTE slavery up or down—to control their own affairs. —That's forgotten now, all that Nebraska flapdoodle and the effigies.

ADELE

Nothing's forgotten, Stephen. You may be the fair-haired
Little Giant to more people now than ever before . . . but nobody's forgotten the riots—nobody's forgotten that a Congress-
man almost beat to death one of your colleagues—right in the
Senate chamber of the United States.

DOUGLAS

No colleague of mine.

ADELE

That doesn't matter! A fellow Senator! Think anybody's forgotten that? And nobody's forgotten that two hundred men,
women and children have been shot and stabbed and burned
to death over this slavery business. Why, their bodies aren't
even cold yet, and here you are going out on a campaign for
re-election to a job in the Senate that nobody on earth could
take away from you if you just made a reasonable, conservative
campaign of it.

DOUGLAS

Just what do you mean by a reasonable conservative campaign? What's wrong with what I'm doing?

ADELE

You're inviting danger, that's what's wrong. I've never heard
of such a thing! Passions are wild enough as it is without your
stepping into a hornet's nest with Lincoln. God knows what
lunatics in a crowd might do . . . and with all these abolitionists
fighting mad about the Dred Scott decision. Don't think Lincoln won't use that against you. He'll throw it at you!

DOUGLAS

Adele, first of all I'm not afraid of lunatics, crowds, effigy-
burners, or fanatic abolitionists. Second, and more important,
I'm afraid of nothing Lincoln may use or throw or say or do.

11

You yourself said he's the best man the Republicans have got.

DOUGLAS

Of all the damned Republican rascals about Springfield, yes, he's the ablest and most honest! But I tell you, the time has not yet come when a handful of Republicans can turn the great State of Illinois into a Negro-worshipping, Negro-equality community. Neither Abe Lincoln nor anyone else!

ADELE

If he gets the better of you in these debates you'll have everything to lose—more than the Senatorship of Illinois, perhaps.

DOUGLAS

Lincoln get the better of me? Is that all the confidence you have in me?

ADELE

I don't trust Republicans!

DOUGLAS

I can handle them. *Including* Abe Lincoln. Adele, my dear, I *know* this man. We opposed each other in the Truett murder trial as long as twenty years ago. When you were still a school child, Abe Lincoln debated me in Bloomington. He was filling in for that idiot Stuart.

ADELE

Isn't Stuart the man you bit on the thumb? Or is he the one you beat with a *cane?*

DOUGLAS

He's lucky he didn't *lose* that thumb. —Well, so I've *already* debated with Lincoln. I licked him all hollow.

ADELE

As you remember it.

DOUGLAS

Adele, are you coming with me or not?

ADELE

No. I've told you that a thousand times, and nothing you can say is going to change my mind. (DOUGLAS *looks at her with quiet admiration, then takes her in his arms and kisses her*)

DOUGLAS

(*Quietly*) I'll tell Elizabeth to get your trunks ready. (HE *leaves her; goes out L.* SHE *looks after him. The* LIGHTING *changes to the reminiscent key.* ADELE *faces the audience*)

ADELE

Of course I went. I always knew I would. It was a grueling campaign. One would think they were running for President, so avid was the interest, so huge the crowds. In seven cities and towns they debated. There were receptions, parades, competing brass bands, fife and drum corps, serenades, saluting cannons. . . . Whenever they appeared on the same platform, people came by the thousands . . . came by train, boat, wagon, some of them walking for miles—to sit or stand in a public square, under a merciless sun, or in a pouring rain, to hear their champions speak. . . . (*As* ADELE *leaves at L, light begins to come up. A fife and drum corps, perhaps a band of the kind Adele has described, is heard banging away. Cannons go off, too—one of them quite close at hand. After a long moment in which the unpopulated stage has come to a full, hot noonday light,* ABRAHAM LINCOLN *enters from R, wearing his stovepipe hat. A partisan band (offstage) hits it up good now, and Lincoln crosses down to the platform, mounts it, takes his hat off, and begins to remove scraps of paper and notes from inside the deep hat—a filing system he often carried around on his*

13

*head. In the progress of getting settled, he drops his watch on
the wooden floor, picks it up, listens to see if it is still running,
then starts to sit when he is distracted by a loud voice at upstage L, behind him. It is the voice of* DOUGLAS, *who has entered, confident and in a jovial mood. He calls offstage to
Adele, as much for the benefit of her friends, as for Adele
herself)*

DOUGLAS

Don't let them keep you from the platform too long, Adele.
. . . They can admire you from a distance. (*He sees Lincoln,
who greets him*)

LINCOLN

Good afternoon, Judge.

DOUGLAS

I'm not late, am I Lincoln?

LINCOLN

No, we still have a minute or two . . . looks like there might
be twenty thousand people out there, Judge.

DOUGLAS

Ah yes, I have quite a number of adherents in this part of
the State.

LINCOLN

(*Amiably*) I'll see what I can do to change that.

DOUGLAS

One can always try. Is Mrs. Lincoln with you?

LINCOLN

No. She doesn't like the smell of gunpowder.

DOUGLAS

I'm sorry. I had hoped to renew an old acquaintance, as well as to hear some of your new stories. What was the one you were telling the boys as we came through?

LINCOLN

(*Starting away*) Oh, that's not much of a story. . . .

DOUGLAS

(*Holding an arm*) Come on, Lincoln.

LINCOLN

(*Making the best of it*) Well, it seems there was an aging father whose son was still a bachelor at the age of 42, and he said to him, "Son—if you want to please yore old paw, you'll take you a wife." "Why sure," answered the son, "just tell me whose wife to take." (DOUGLAS *laughs a little too heartily for the speed of the joke*) Well, it's not *that* good. . . .

DOUGLAS

(*Not to be outdone*) Lincoln . . . have you heard the story of the itinerant preacher and the chimpanzee? (*Looks around to make sure nobody will overhear. Then he turns his back to the audience and tells the story into the big left ear of Lincoln, who stoops forward to hear it. As Lincoln is standing on the speaking platform and Douglas on the raked stage, the already marked difference in height between the two men, is further accentuated. When Douglas finishes the story, Lincoln rears back in hilarious laughter.* DOUGLAS, *having made a success with his presumably shady story, quits when he is ahead, and darts toward the upper L corner to escort* ADELE, *who has just entered*) Adele . . . darling . . . (*He gallantly escorts her to her chair on the speaking platform.* LINCOLN, *still quaking with laughter from Douglas's story, cannot quite assume the dignity and gravity that would be appropriate for the moment when his opponent's wife enters the scene . . . and* ADELE, *for her*

15

part, wonders what manner of buffoon her husband has gotten involved with. She looks quizzically at DOUGLAS, *as though to say, "What's the matter with him?" But* DOUGLAS *gives her a reassuring nod, and both sit in their respective chairs.* LINCOLN *and* DOUGLAS *wait for a moment, as though for the audience to settle; then* LINCOLN *rises*)

LINCOLN

(*Still hungover from the amusement*) When I was a boy, I spent considerable time on the Sangamon River. An old steamboat plied on the river, the boiler of which was so small that when they blew the whistle, there wasn't enough steam to turn the paddle wheel. When the paddle wheel went round, they couldn't blow the whistle. —Now a good many people who argue about slavery, remind me of that old steamboat—when they talk they can't think, and when they think they can't talk. —I will try not to be like them. (DOUGLAS *chuckles. Now* LINCOLN *gets down to business*) Fellow citizens: I wish to make a distinction between the existing institution of slavery and the extension of it, so broad and so clear, that no honest man can misunderstand me, and no dishonest one misrepresent me. When Southern people tell us they are no more responsible for the origin of slavery than we are, I acknowledge the fact. When it is said that the institution exists, and is very difficult to get rid of in any satisfactory way, I can understand and appreciate the saying. But the opening of new territories to slavery tends to its perpetuation, and so keeps men in slavery who would otherwise be free. Justice to the South, they tell us, requires us to consent to the extension of slavery to new territories. That is to say, inasmuch as you don't object to my taking my hog to Nebraska, therefore I mustn't object to your taking your slave. I admit that this is perfectly logical, if there's no difference between hogs and negroes. Now, Thomas Jefferson, the author of the Declaration of Independence, conceived of the policy of prohibiting slavery in new territory. Thus, away back in the pure, fresh, free breath of the Revolution, Congress put that policy in practice. (*Turning to look at* DOUGLAS) But now, new light breaks upon us. We find some men, who drew every breath of their lives under this very restriction, who now live in dread of absolute suffocation, if they should be restricted in the sacred right of taking slaves to the new territory of Nebraska. That perfect Liberty they sigh for—the liberty of making slaves of other people—Jefferson never thought of; their own fathers never thought of; they never thought of it *themselves,* a year ago! How fortunate for them they did not sooner become sensible of their great misery!

DOUGLAS

(*Rising*) May I have a word, Mr. Lincoln?

LINCOLN

You may, Judge.

DOUGLAS

(*To Audience*) Mr. Lincoln is saying that when our fathers made this government, they never thought of the state of things now existing. Well, they never thought of the telegraph that transmits intelligence by lightning; they never thought of the railroads; so let's not bewail everything our fathers never thought of, including the thousand mechanical inventions that have elevated mankind. (*Sits*)

LINCOLN

(*Resuming*) I'm for elevating mankind, too. . . . But this zeal for the spread of slavery, I cannot but hate. I hate it because of the monstrous injustice of slavery itself. I hate it because it deprives our republican example of its just influence in the world; enables the enemies of free institutions to taunt us with justice as hypocrites; causes the real friends of freedom to doubt our sincerity; and especially because it forces so many really good men among ourselves into an open war with the fundamental principles of civil liberty. Before proceeding, let me say I have no prejudice against the Southern people. The great majority South, as well as North, have human sympathies, of which they can no more divest themselves, than they can of their sensibility to physical pain. If they deny this, let me address them one plain question: There are in the United States 433,000 free blacks. At $500 a head, they're worth over two hundred millions of dollars! How comes this vast amount of property to be running about, without owners? All these free blacks would be *slaves,* but for something which has operated on their white owners, inducing them at vast pecuniary sacrifices to *liberate* them. What is that something? Is there any mistaking it? It is their sense of justice and human sympathy, continually telling them that the poor Negro has some natural right to himself—that these who deny it, and make mere merchandise of him, deserve kickings, contempt and death!

DOUGLAS
(*Angrily*) Mr. Lincoln. . . . I must call your attention to the incontestable fact that—

LINCOLN
(*Cutting him off*) Just a moment—

DOUGLAS
(*Riding over him*) —some of the finest people in this country—

LINCOLN
(*Firmly*) There is one more point I would like to make before I'm through.

DOUGLAS
(*Snapping*) Well, kindly make it, sir! (HE *looks at Adele, righteously*)

LINCOLN
You may rest assured that I will.

DOUGLAS
Very well. (*taking his own sweet time,* LINCOLN *picks up a glass of water, drinks it, looks at his watch, resumes:*)

LINCOLN

I want to take up the case of Dred Scott—the slave who sued for freedom because he was taken into territory where slavery is illegal. The decision of the United States Supreme Court declares in effect that a Negro is property, and if a slave-owner takes him to free territory, that property can't be taken from him. The decision reads that Negroes—quote—"Had for more than a century been regarded as beings of an inferior order, altogether unfit to associate with the white race; and so *far* inferior that they had no rights which the white man was bound to respect; and that the Negro might justly and lawfully be reduced to slavery for his *benefit.*" I am still quoting from the Supreme Court of the United States. The decision goes on to quote from the Declaration of Independence that all men are created equal, and *adds* in these words: "But it is too clear for dispute, that the enslaved African race *were not intended to be included.*" Now that decision was made by a court divided 6 to 2. Judge Douglas here denounces all who question that decision, as offering violent resistance to it. But who *resists* it? Who, has, in spite of it, *freed* Dred Scott? I believe as much as Judge Douglas—perhaps more—in obedience to the court. I think its decisions, when fully settled, should control not only the particular cases but the general policy of the country. But I think the Dred Scott decision is *erroneous!* The court that made it has often overruled its own decisions, and we shall do what we can to have it overrule *this!* (HE *sits.* DOUGLAS *rises, grim and determined. He has the air of a man about to demolish a fractious opponent*)

DOUGLAS

In Mr. Lincoln's ecstasy over the wrongs of the Dred Scott decision, he makes a great parade of his hatred for slavery. But he chose not to tell you one significant thing. You will find he has a fertile genius for concealing his thoughts when it serves him to do so. Mr. Lincoln chose not to tell you that at the time the case went to the Supreme Court, Dred Scott was a slave owned by one of Mr. Lincoln's friends—an abolitionist member of Congress from Springfield, Massachusetts.

LINCOLN

I never pretended to know whether Dred Scott's owners were Democrats or Abolitionists or border ruffians. I don't see that it matters.

DOUGLAS

He doesn't see. —It matters, sir, because so many Abolitionists pretend horror at the bondage of the slave, and yet they enjoy the benefits of slavery.—*That's* why it matters. (*Squarely to audience*) Now my fellow citizens: As a *lawyer*, I feel at liberty to appear before the Supreme Court and controvert any principle of the law while the question is pending before the tribunal. But when the decision is made, my private opinion, *your* opinion, all *other* opinions, must yield to the majesty of the authoritative adjudication. I wish you to bear in mind, my friends, that this involves a great principle, upon which our rights, our liberty, and our property all depend. (*To* LINCOLN) What security have you for your property, your reputation, and your personal rights, if the courts are not upheld, and their decisions respected?

LINCOLN

The sacredness that you throw around this decision has never been thrown around any other. It is the first of its kind; an astonisher in legal history; a new wonder of the world.

DOUGLAS

Yes . . . well, I will get back to Mr. Lincoln's darling project of overriding the Supreme Court in another moment—but first I'd like to chase a certain notion out of his troubled brain.

20

When the Declaration of Independence was put forth, every
one of the thirteen colonies was slave-holding, and every man
who signed the instrument, represented a slave-holding con-
stituency! *Not one* of them freed his slaves, much less put them
on an equality with himself, *after* he signed the Declaration.
Now, Mr. Lincoln instructs us that the Declaration means the
Negro to be the equal of the white man. Are you willing to have
it said that every man who signed that instrument believing the
Negro to be his equal, was a hypocrite? Are you charging the
signers of our Declaration with *hypocrisy?*

LINCOLN

You've got it all wrong, Judge. I would remind you of
Thomas Jefferson's words on the subject of slavery. He said,
"I tremble for my country when I remember that God is just."
—I will offer the highest premium in my power to Judge Doug-
las if he will show that in all his life he ever uttered a sentiment
at all akin to that.

DOUGLAS

If God ever intended the Negro to be the equal of the white
man, He has been a long time in demonstrating that fact.

LINCOLN

So now Judge Douglas is arguing with the Almighty as well
as with Thomas Jefferson.

DOUGLAS

(*With mock weariness*) Aaaah, Thomas Jefferson again!
May I remind you that Mr. Jefferson was a slave-holder all his
life!

LINCOLN

That argument is just about as thin as the soup that was
made by boiling the shadow of a pigeon that starved to death.
Contrary to your fond recollection, Mr. Jefferson and the fathers
of our country did *not* make this nation part slave and part

free. They *found* the institution of slavery already in existence. They did not *make* it so. And the only reason they *left* it so, was because they knew of no way to get rid of it at that time.

DOUGLAS

(*Disgusted*) Hah!

LINCOLN

So when you ask me why our government can't remain as our fathers made it, I turn around and ask you the same question.

DOUGLAS

Ask that question of the Supreme Court, sir!

LINCOLN

I have done so, and will continue to do so.

DOUGLAS

Ah yes, so you have. Well—by now we may safely assume that Mr. Lincoln is opposed to the Dred Scott decision. All right, suppose he is; what's he going to do about it? I never got beat in a law suit in my life, that I wasn't opposed to the decision. He says he won't fight the judges in order to liberate Dred Scott, but that he will not respect that decision as a rule of law binding on this country. Why not? —Because, he says, it's unjust. How's he going to remedy it? He's going to *reverse* it. —How? —He's going to take an appeal. —To *whom* is he going to appeal? —Why, he's going to appeal to the people to elect a new president who will appoint judges who will *reverse* that decision. Well, let's see HOW that's going to be done. The only way it can be done is to carry on until he gets a Republican president elected. —*AND I DON'T BELIEVE HE EVER WILL!* (HE *sits, well pleased with himself.* LINCOLN *rises*)

LINCOLN

Well, circumstances alter cases.

22

Certainly do!

You remember we once had a national bank. Some one owed
the bank a debt; he was sued, and sought to avoid payment on
the ground that the bank was unconstitutional. The case went
to the Supreme Court, which decided that the bank *was* constitutional. Judge Douglas' Democratic Party revolted against that
decision. President Jackson himself vetoed a charter for the
bank. —I have heard Judge Douglas say that he *approved* of
President Jackson for that act. —So what has now become of
all his tirade about resistance to the Supreme Court? The plain
truth is simply this: Judge Douglas is *for* Supreme Court decisions when he likes them; and *against* them when he doesn't
like them.

(*Remaining seated*) I don't choose to continue any argument
to prove that the Justices of the Supreme Court understand law
better than Abe Lincoln. —What he's saying is that *I* am *bound*
by Supreme Court decisions, and *he* is *not.* (*To Lincoln*) You
should know better than to try to palm off such vulgar imposi-
tions upon this extremely intelligent audience!

May I remind the Judge of another piece of history on the
question of respect for judicial decisions: A piece of *Illinois*
history belonging to a time when Judge Douglas was displeased
with a decision of the Supreme Court of Illinois. Then he was
in favor of overturning that decision by the device of adding
five new judges, so as to vote down the four-old ones! Not only
that, but it ended in the Judge here sitting down on that very
bench AS one of the five new judges to break down the four
old ones! And it was in this way precisely that he got his title
of Judge. Now, when *he* tells *me* that men appointed to sit as
members of a court will have to be catechized beforehand upon

some subject, I say, "You *know*, Judge; you have tried it."
—When he imputes that a court of this kind will lose the confidence of all men, will be prostituted and disgraced by such a proceeding, I say, "You know best, Judge; you have been through the mill." (HE *sits.* DOUGLAS *rises, pale with indignation, very grave*)

DOUGLAS

Forgive me if, on this occasion, I do not participate in Mr. Lincoln's celebrated humor. —I see nothing funny in his attempt to bring the Supreme Court into disrepute. He is willing to destroy public confidence in the highest judicial tribunal on earth, simply because it does not put the Negro on an equality with the white man. Well, let me make this clear. I am *opposed* to Negro equality! This nation is a nation of white people of European descent: a people that have established this government for themselves and their posterity—and I am in favor of preserving not only the purity of government, but the purity of *blood* from any mixtures with inferior races! I am opposed to taking any step which recognizes the Negro or the Indian as the *equal* of the White Man! Now, I would extend to the Negro, and to the Indian, and to all dependent races every right, every privilege, every immunity consistent with the safety and welfare of the white races; but *equality* they *never* should have, either political, or social, or in any other respect whatever. Each state must decide for *itself* the nature and extent of these rights. Illinois has decided for herself that the Negro shall *not* vote, or serve on juries, or enjoy political privileges. I am content with that system. I deny the right of any other state to complain of our policy, or attempt to change it. On the other hand, the state of Maine has decided that in that state a Negro man may vote on an equality with the white man. Maine has the *right* to prescribe that rule for herself. New York has decided that a Negro may vote, provided he owns $250 worth of property, but not otherwise. The rich Negro can vote, but the poor one cannot. Although that distinction does not com-

mend itself to my judgment, New York has a *right* to prescribe
that form of the elective franchise. I do *not* acknowledge that
the Negro must have civil and political rights everywhere or
nowhere. Thus you see, my fellow-citizens, that the issues between Mr. Lincoln and myself, as respective candidates for the
United States Senate, are direct, unequivocal, and irreconcila-
ble! (LIGHT FADES TO BLACKOUT. *In the interval, a band comes
out on the forestage and plays a spanking tune of the period.
When it leaves and the* LIGHT *comes up again, it is a warm
summer night and the* DOUGLASES *are on the porch of a hotel
. . . indicated only by a wicker chair at extreme lower R.* ADELE
is fanning herself; DOUGLAS *is pacing behind her. With her
back to him, and his to her,* DOUGLAS *reaches inside his coat
pocket for a flask which he just starts to drink from when:*)

ADELE

(*Face still front; without changing expression*) It gurgles—
Stephen, put it away.

DOUGLAS

Just soothing my tonsils. They get raw out there on the
platform.

ADELE

(*Not unsympathically*) I'm sure.

DOUGLAS

(*Sitting beside her*) Is something worrying you?

ADELE

Certainly not. What makes you think that I'm worried?

DOUGLAS

The way you waggle that fan.

ADELE

It's a hot night, that's all.

DOUGLAS

I'm sure. —I tell you, if it keeps up, this agitation is going to split the country in two. What do they think I'm shouting about? I want to preserve the Union! . . . to keep it from breaking up over this damned nonsensical slavery issue! If we're not careful this Black Republican—you're not listening, Adele.

ADELE

Stephen: Do you think it's wise for us to travel in a private railway car all through the campaign? With that brass cannon on your flatcar shooting off at every stop? Some people are horrified at the extravagance of it.

DOUGLAS

Only Republicans—and they're horrified at everything. Except Negro equality.

ADELE

Even one of our own people raised an eyebrow today.

DOUGLAS

Who?

ADELE

I've forgotten his name. He was in the local delegation.

DOUGLAS

What did he say?

ADELE

He said the Republicans are making capital of the lie that the railroad has given us the car free.

DOUGLAS

(*Laughs*) Did you tell him that would be like getting whiskey from the udder of a cow?

No. —What I told him was that a private railway car is a way of saving your strength and health in an extremely rigorous campaign. I said that the car gives you a place to receive newspapermen and local delegations. Also, I said, it's good showmanship.

Was he impressed?

Not by that so much as by my pointing out that in addition to the seven joint debates, you're scheduled to make 59 speeches in 57 counties, each from two to three hours in in length—and God knows how many *impromptu* speeches you'll have to make. I told him you'll be traveling over 5000 miles attending receptions, arranging finances, and trying to keep peace among grumbling party workers like himself.

(*Jumps up; disturbed*) Did you say that? "Grumbling"?

(*Enjoying her joke*) No. I said "honestly perturbed."

(*Relaxing*) Adele, you're a genius.

Well, the man was all choked up by the time I was through. I left him thinking you were just about the greatest thing that ever walked the soil of his sacred Illinois.

(*Admiringly*) How can I lose, Adele, how can I lose?

ADELE

(*Earnestly; as she starts to exit at R*) Easily, Stephen—by being careless.

DOUGLAS

(*Calling after her*) You worry about the damndest things.

ADELE

(*Almost off*) I'm a woman. . . . (*As they both leave, a* REPUBLICAN COMMITTEEMAN *enters from R. He is a bustling and bumbling type, not much accustomed to public speaking, bue he rather enjoys the little moment of glory this gives him, and this partly overcomes his sense of inadequacy as a forceful politico*)

REPUBLICAN COMMITTEEMAN

(*Addressing the audience*) Begging your indulgence please. . . . I have a few announcements for fellow Republicans in this gathering. As you know, Judge Douglas, the political knave and demagogue, is being met tomorrow by a torchlite procession of his worshippers—with transparencies, music, cannons, and live Democrats—and it is up to us to go them one better! Now Lincoln, the Champion of Freedom, is coming in with the Knoxville delegation and will be met by our escort of honor consisting of citizens on foot one mile from the square. The Abingdon delegation will be on the 10 o'clock train . . . Oneida and Wataga delegations on the 11. An excursion train will come over the Peoria and Oquawka line arriving at noon, at reduced rates. The ladies, God bless 'em, are invited to grace the proceedings with their presence. Special roomy carriages will be loaded with the fair freight. Let us all turn out to support the Tall Sucker against the so-called Little Giant, who is as much a blackguard as he is a demagogue, and scarcely has an equal in either respect. In fact, bad whiskey and the wear and tear of conscience are showing their effect on him. Thank you for your kind and gracious indulgence. (HE *scrambles off R. In the half light still left over from this vignette, the*

-28

DOUGLASES *and* LINCOLN *take their positions on the platform, the* DOUGLASES *sitting on their chairs.* LINCOLN *starts to speak simultaneously with the rise of light to full, hot, debating strength*)

LINCOLN

Judge Douglas has the high distinction, so far as I know, of never having said slavery is either right or wrong. Everybody else says one thing or the other, but the Judge never does. My friends, our Declaration of Independence was thought to include all; but now, to aid in making the bondage of the Negro universal and eternal, it is assailed, and sneered at, and construed, and hawked at, and torn, till, if its framers could rise from their graves, they could not at all recognize it. All the powers on earth seem rapidly combining against the Negro. The God of money is after him; ambition follows; philosophy follows; and the theology of the day is fast joining the cry. They have him in his prisonhouse; they have searched his person and left no prying instruments with him. One after another they have closed the heavy iron doors upon him; and now they have him, as it were, bolted-in with a lock of a hundred keys, which can never be unlocked without the concurrence of every key; the keys in the hands of a hundred different men, and they scattered to a hundred different and distant places; and they stand *musing* as to what invention, in all the dominions of mind and matter, can be procured to make the impossibility of his escape more complete than it is. Certainly the Negro is not our equal in color—perhaps not in many other respects; still, in the right to put into his mouth the bread that his own hands have earned, he is my equal, the equal of Judge Douglas, the equal of every living man, white or black! In pointing out that more has been given you, you cannot be justified in taking away the little that has been given him. All I ask for the Negro is that if you don't like him, let him alone! If God gave him but little, that little let him enjoy! Go ahead, Judge Douglas. (HE *sits*)

29

DOUGLAS

(*Almost contemptuously*) A very moving speech, Mr. Lincoln. (*Rises; gravely*) But the perils of our problem are such that they will not permit of easy sentiment or grieving hearts. Please—let us cling to the *issues!* I will be entirely frank with you. I deny the right of Congress to force a slave-holding state upon an unwilling people. I deny their right to force a *free* state upon an unwilling people. I deny their right to force a good thing upon a people who are unwilling to receive it. The great principle is the right of every community to decide for *itself* whether a thing is right or wrong, whether it would be good or evil for them to adopt it; and the right of free action, the right of free thought, is dearer to every true American than any other under a free government. It is no answer to this argument to say that slavery is an evil, and hence should not be tolerated. You must allow the people to *decide for themselves* whether it is good or evil. You allow them to decide for themselves what kind of schools they will have; what system of banking they will adopt; you allow them to decide for themselves the relations between husband and wife, parent and child, guardian and ward—in fact, you allow them to decide for themselves all *other* questions; why not THIS question?! (*With a tone of warning*) Once you put a limitation upon the right of any people to decide what laws they want, you have destroyed the fundamental principle of self-government! My friends, who among us expects to live or have his children live, until slavery shall be abolished in South Carolina or established in Illinois? Who expects to see that occur during the lifetime of ourselves or our children? There is but one possible way in which slavery can be abolished, and that is by leaving a state perfectly free to regulate its institutions *in its own way!* That was the principle upon which this Republic was founded; and under its operations, slavery *disappeared* from *six* of the twelve original slave-holding States! This gradual system of emancipation went on quietly, peacefully, and steadily, so long as the Free States minded their own business and left their neighbors alone; but

30

the moment the North said: "We are powerful enough to control you of the South"; the moment the North proclaimed itself the determined *master* of the South, that moment the South combined to *resist* the attack, and thus sectional parties were formed and gradual emancipation *ceased* in all the Northern slaveholding states! Now friend Lincoln wants his colored brethren to vote. If they had a vote, I reckon they would all vote for *him* in preference to *me,* entertaining the views I do. But that matters not. The position he has taken not only claims for the Negro the right to vote, but the right, under the divine law, to be elected to office, to become members of the Legislature, to go to Congress, to become Governors, or United States Senators, or Judges of the Supreme Court; and I suppose that when they *control* that court, they will probably reverse the Dred Scott decision. Well, I confess to you, I am utterly opposed to that! The signers of the Declaration never supposed it *possible* that their language would be *used* in an attempt to make this nation a mixed nation of Indians, Negroes, Whites and Mongrels! (*Sits*)

LINCOLN

(*Rising*) As a nation we began by declaring that all men are created equal. We now practically read it, "All men are created equal except Negroes." When the Know-Nothings get control it will read, "All men are created equal except Negroes, and foreigners, and Catholics." When it comes to this I should prefer emigrating to some country where they make no pretense of loving liberty . . . some country like Russia, where despotism can be taken pure without the base alloy of hypocrisy.(*Having purged himself of his anger in the foregoing, he regains some of his humor, and takes on a pleasantly foxy look*) Now Judge Douglas boldly denies that the Declaration of Independence includes Negroes at *all,* and proceeds to argue gravely that all who contend it does, do so only because they want to vote, and eat, and sleep with, and marry Negroes. Well, I protest against the counterfeit logic which concludes that, because I do not

want a black woman for a slave, I must necessarily want her
for a wife. I have lived nearly half a century without having
had her for either. We can leave one another alone and do one
another much good thereby. There are white men enough to
marry all the white women, and enough black men to marry all
the black women; and in God's name let them be so married!
I have never had the least apprehension that I or my friends
would marry Negroes if there was no law to keep us from it;
but as Judge Douglas and his friends seem to be worried that
they might, if there were no law to keep them from it, I give
him the most solemn pledge that I will stand by the law which
forbids it. I will add one further word, which is this: there is
no place where the relations of the Negro and the white man
can be altered except here at home in the state legislature, and
not in Washington.—

DOUGLAS

(*Rising*) That's right!

LINCOLN

And as Judge Douglas seems to be in constant horror that
some such danger is rapidly approaching, I propose as the best
means to prevent it, that the Judge be *kept here at home,* and
placed in the State Legislature to *fight* the measure!

DOUGLAS

Where the people of Illinois wish to place me, Mr. Lincoln,
will soon be manifest. I suspect that it will be at a sufficient
distance from your accustomed haunts in Illinois, that you will
from time to time grow lonely for me.

LINCOLN

Not likely, Judge.

DOUGLAS

Obviously, Mr. Lincoln wishes to confer upon the Negro
all the rights of citizens. I won't quarrel with him for his views
on that subject. —But ask any of those gallant young men

who went to Mexico to fight and die in the battles of their
country (in what friend Lincoln considered an unjust and unholy war), and hear what they will tell you in regard to the
amalgamation of races in that country. Is it not true, Mr. Lincoln, that amalgamation there has reduced that mongrel people
below the capacity of self-government?

LINCOLN

We are not discussing—

DOUGLAS

(*Turning his back on him*) Fellow-citizens, I appeal to your
judgment to approve or disapprove *my* principles, as com-
pared with those of Mr. Lincoln. I am aware that this is a
bitter and severe contest, but I do not doubt what your decision
will be. I don't anticipate any personnel collision between Mr.
Lincoln and myself. He is a fine lawyer, he possesses high
ability, and there is no objection to him—*except the monstrous
revolutionary doctrines with which he is identified and is
determined to carry out if he gets the power!* One more point.
—The Republican leaders have formed an alliance against me—
an unholy, unnatural alliance—with a portion of unscrupulous
Democrat officeholders. I intend to fight that allied army whenever I meet them. (*Forcefully*) I shall deal with these allied
forces just as the Russians dealt with the Allies at Sebastopol
in the late Crimean War. The Russians, defending Sebastopol,
when they fired a broadside at the common enemy, did not
stop to inquire whether it hit a Frenchman, an Englishman, or
a Turk—nor will *I* stop to inquire whether *my* blows hit the
Republican-leaders or their Democrat allies!

LINCOLN

(*Having fun*) Just think of it! Judge Douglas is the rugged
Russian Bear! If there *is* such an alliance as he says there is—
that some of the administration men and we Republicans are
allied, and stand in the attitude of the English, French and

33

Turk, he occupying the position of the Russian—in that case, I beg that he will indulge me while I barely suggest to him that those allies *took* Sebastopol! (BLACKOUT. *As the principals exit,* DOUGLAS *R and* LINCOLN *L, a spot comes up on a* LADY DOUGLASITE *who enters from downstage R*)

A LADY DOUGLASITE

Sister Democrats and Ladies: You will be pleased to know that the Carroll County Women for Douglas are with you of Winnebago one hundred percent in this canvas. I have been asked by the Chairlady of our group to introduce to you a song written for our candidate by a gentleman from Galesboro. —Now, I am not a singer, just a loyal Douglasite, but my group thinks you ought to hear the words and melody so you can all go out and sing it where it will do the most good. It is called HURRAH HURRAH FROM HILL AND VALLEY and has three verses. I will do the best I can to stay on key without a pianist to accompany me. (*Singing*)

> Hurrah Hurrah from hill and valley
> Hurrah from prairie wide and free
> Around our glorious leader rally
> For Douglas and Democracy.
>
> We won't vote for Lincoln; he is not our man
> We'll stick to brave Douglas as long as we can.
>
> Though Lincoln oppose him he surely will yield
> And Stephen A. Douglas will conquer the field.
> Hurrah for our leader, long may he be
> *Senator* Douglas for you and for me!

I think it has lasting value. Other verses will be written if need be. I hope you like it enough to sing it up and down the length and breadth of the county, and across the prairie wide and free. Thank you. (*She exits R. Now we discover* ADELE *at upper Stage R; she is dressed for travel. Under the following speech (but not before)* LINCOLN *is discovered at L sitting in a vintage train coach chair, working on some writing. A carpet bag rests on the floor by the side of the chair; his tall silk hat rests, open side up, on the seat next to him)*

ADELE

(*Coming forward*) At every stop along the way I attended receptions to lady Democrats. Once my husband had gone on ahead to a meeting and I was riding on a train to join him. To my surprise I found that Abraham Lincoln was in the car— and the only empty seat was next to his. My first thought was that it would be disloyal to sit next to him. Then I thought it would be disloyal to *not* sit next to him. (*She crosses to the seat; LINCOLN rises when HE sees her*)

LINCOLN

Mrs. Douglas! —What a pleasure to see you outside of the arena!

ADELE

Thank you, Mr. Lincoln. —Is it all right to sit here, or should I be afraid of you?

LINCOLN

Madam, your relationship with the Senator gives you very special immunities. (*Indicating the chair*) Please . . . (ADELE *lifts the hat from the chair and hands it to* LINCOLN)

ADELE

You wouldn't want me to crush your hat. Not even my husband has rained blows that hard on your head.

LINCOLN

(*Laughing*) Hard enough. (THEY *sit; for a moment there is an awkward pause*)

LINCOLN

That reminds me of the man who was sitting in the theater, and there was an empty seat beside him, on which he placed his tall silk hat—open side up. Well, he was busy watching the play, and he didn't notice a stout woman come in and sit beside him. In the dark she didn't see the hat, and she sat down heavily. There was a loud crunch, and the woman shot up immediately. The man reached for his flattened hat, took one look at it, and said, "Madam, I could have *told* you my hat wouldn't fit you before you tried it on." (ADELE *only smiles*) I hope you didn't mind that.

ADELE

Not at all. I've heard a great deal of your reputation as a teller of stories, and I am glad to have had the rumor demonstrated and confirmed.

LINCOLN

Well, I suppose some of the stories aren't so nice as they might be, but I tell you the truth when I say that a good story, if it has the element of genuine wit, has the same effect on me that I suppose a good square drink of whiskey has on an old toper: it puts new life into me. I sometimes use jokes to cure my own blues; sometimes to clinch an argument, or disarm an antagonist. A good story can be a sort of labor-saving device.

ADELE

You realize you're giving secrets to the enemy?

LINCOLN

A calculated risk and a welcome one, ma'am.

ADELE

You're very gallant. I think you would make an excellent Senator, Mr. Lincoln—although you'll understand if I say not quite as excellent as the *incumbent.*

LINCOLN

(*Laughing*) Well, Im convinced that I'm good enough for it; but in spite of it all, I say to myself every day, "It's too big a thing for you—you'll never get it." —Don't let the Judge quote that against me, now.

36

Not even the Judge's wife will. —What does Mrs. Lincoln think? Does she share your views as partisanly as I do my husband's?

LINCOLN

Oh, I guess so. I tried out some logic on her a while back, and she thought it was the greatest thing since the invention of fire. It was sort of a mathematical formula on the slavery issue.

ADELE

That sounds intriguing. If it wouldn't be divulging strategy that my husband's chief spy can use, would you care to try it out on me?

LINCOLN

Oh, it's a simple enough hypothesis. It's like this: If A can prove, however conclusively, that he has a right to enslave B, why may not B snatch the same argument, and prove equally that he has a right to enslave A?

ADELE

Well—because A is white and B is black.

LINCOLN

It's color, then? The lighter having the right to enslave the darker? —Take care. By this rule, you'd be a slave to the first person you meet with a fairer skin than your own.

ADELE

Well, I didn't mean *color* exactly. I mean that the whites are *intellectually* the superiors of the blacks.

LINCOLN

Take care again. By this rule you'd be slave to the first person you meet with an *intellect* superior to your own.

ADELE

But it's a question of *interest,* isn't it?

37

LINCOLN

You mean if you can make it your *interest*, you have the right
to enslave another? (SHE *does not answer*) By the same token,
if he can make it *his* interest he has the right to enslave *you.*

ADELE

Oh dear, I really should leave this sort of thing to my husband.

LINCOLN

I'd a lot rather he left it to you.

ADELE

(*Smiling*) Thank you. (*Looking out of the imaginary window*) We're almost there, aren't we?

LINCOLN

Yes, ma'am.

ADELE

Tell me something, Mr. Lincoln, before we part—there has
been a great deal of angry name-calling in the press on both
sides. We get newspaper clippings from friends all over the
country. How do you keep your temper when someone pub-
lishes a full-blown lie about you?

LINCOLN

Ah, Mrs. Douglas, if one were to run down all the insinua-
tions, inveracities and innuendoes uttered against a man in
public, life would be nothing but a perpetual flea hunt.

ADELE

"Perpetual flea hunt." Very good.

LINCOLN

(*Rising*) And here we are. I suppose I lose you to my worthy
opponent now?

ADELE

(*Rising also*) He'll be here to meet me. —What do you suppose he'll say about our having exchanged notes?

LINCOLN

Whatever he says, I'll rebutt it. (HE *takes her arm and leads her to R.* DOUGLAS *emerges from the wings and expresses amiable surprise when* HE *sees her with* LINCOLN) Judge Douglas, here's your good woman that I brought along. She can do more with you than I can.

DOUGLAS

(*With mock dismay*) Archangels and archenemies together!

LINCOLN

I told her everything I know. It didn't take long.

ADELE

I've been doing a little reconnoitering for you, Stephen. Now you'll be able to match him story for story.

DOUGLAS

It would take more than a little reconnoitering. —Coming our way, Lincoln?

LINCOLN

No thanks, I'll have my own conveyance. —See you at the barricades, Judge. You too, Mrs. Douglas.

DOUGLAS

Good day. (THEY *wave each other a cordial goodbye; the* DOUGLASES *exit R;* LINCOLN, *after a moment in which he watches them go off, turns and leaves in the opposite direction. The light fades as he crosses, and by the time he passes from view, the stage is dark*)

END OF ACT I

39

ACT TWO

The lights come UP *to discover* DOUGLAS *D.R. seated at a table, making notes on a speech. A bottle of whiskey is at his side. He uncorks the bottle, takes a nip, puts it back, returns to his writing. From offstage comes the* VOICE *of* ADELE.

ADELE

(*Offstage*) Stephen. . . .

DOUGLAS

Yes, dear. . . .

ADELE

(*Still off*) Is it going to take another hour to nudge and squeeze our way through the crowds again today before we get to the platform?

DOUGLAS

I rather like big crowds . . . especially as most of them have been coming out to hear me. . . .

ADELE

(*Entering L; she is sewing a button on Stephen's vest*) All right . . . I don't mind the crowds so much. . . . I don't mind the dreadful bands, or the fireworks, or the 32 girls dressed in white, each bearing the name of a State, with wreaths of prairie flowers—I can put up with the satin banners and the bunting, and the barouches—

DOUGLAS

And the drunk skunk who threw the watermelon rind at me?

40

ADELE

I can be calm about the committees and politicians and advisors, and the yokels who come up spitting tobacco juice and looking at you out of the sides of their eyes because they want to get a peep at a famous man—that's all part of the game—but what I *cannot abide* are gigantic floats that have nothing to do with Democrats or Republicans, but which simply *ADVERTISE* the *George W. Fruehoffer Corn Plaster Works.* (*Bites the thread in two*) What's happened to politics in this country?

DOUGLAS

(*Laughing*) You *do* worry about the damndest things.

ADELE

And that miserable jingle on that great big banner: "THE GIRLS LINK ON TO LINCOLN AS THEIR MOTHERS CLUNG TO CLAY."

DOUGLAS

It never changes. . . . (SHE *crosses to him, hands him the vest, puts her hands on his shoulders, asks earnestly:*)

ADELE

(*Helping him on with the vest*) Stephen—will you think me a bit of a shrew if I pick on you a little? Just about a couple of things?

DOUGLAS

(*Covering her hands with his own*) I'd sooner be henpecked by you than petted by the Queen of Sheba.

ADELE

When that newspaper reporter asked you about the tariff, why did you slough him off?

DOUGLAS

Slough him off? I did no such thing.

41

ADELE

(*Picks up his whiskey bottle, marks the level of the liquor with a pencil*) Do you remember what you said?

DOUGLAS

I don't cling to every word I've said to every reporter who comes up out of the floor to fire questions at me.

ADELE

I remember *exactly*.

DOUGLAS

What did I say?

ADELE

(*Imitating his manner*) What you said was, "My dear fellow, I have learned enough about the tariff to know that I scarcely know anything about it at all; and a man makes considerable *progress* on a question of this kind when he ascertains that fact."

DOUGLAS

(*Chuckling*) Well, what's wrong with that? I thought that was a *good* answer. At least it was honest.

ADELE

Save your good answers for Mr. Lincoln. He nipped you today in the newspaper.

DOUGLAS

How?

ADELE

For your dig at him to the crowd around the train. When you said he once ran a grocery store and sold whiskey.

42

DOUGLAS

Well, so he did.

ADELE

Implying that he's in favor of drinking.

DOUGLAS

Well, what's this about the newspaper?

ADELE

(*Holding up the bottle*) He's reported as saying that the difference between him and you, is that while he was *behind* a bar, you were in *front* of it.

DOUGLAS

(*Laughing; as* HE *rises*) Let him have his jokes. If there's anybody who hugs a flask—

ADELE

Never mind, darling. Just don't do and say impetuous things. Abe Lincoln is no clown, and he has a good chance of beating you in spite of what all your well-wishers and flatterers tell you.

DOUGLAS

I've got something to tell *you!* Do you know Major Stuart has come out for me?

ADELE

(*Shrieking with laughter*) What? The man whose thumb you nearly bit off?

DOUGLAS

It's apparently healed at last.

ADELE

Oh, that's wonderful!

43

DOUGLAS

He was Lincoln's first law partner, too. He announced that on the slavery issue he agrees with *me*—he's wholly opposed to the Republican party. Also, my love, do you know what the betting is?

ADELE

I don't care what the betting is.

DOUGLAS

Well, *I'd* like to do a bit of reading. (*Getting a clipping from the table*) You collect newspaper clippings . . . here's one I'll warrant you didn't see; from Chicago . . .: (*Reading*) "We are authorized to announce that a gentleman of this city would bet $10,000 that Stephen A. Douglas will be re-elected to the Senate of the United States. Come, gentlemen Republicans, show your faith in Abe."

. ADELE

(*Starting off*) All right, let me read something to *you* from the Chicago press.

DOUGLAS

(*Interested*) Oh? What?

ADELE

(*As* SHE *goes through the L door*) You'll see.

DOUGLAS

(*To himself, with a chuckle*) My little filing secretary. . . .

ADELE

(*Returns with a batch of clippings and starts to read them as she crosses*) Listen to this: "Lincoln Wiped Up the Ground With the Little Giant. At the End of the Speech, Douglas Fled, a Defeated Man."

DOUGLAS

(*Nettled*) The swine!

ADELE

(*Another clipping*) The Quincy Whig: "Douglas Actually Foamed at the Mouth." (DOUGLAS *makes a grab for the rest of the clippings in her hands. As he does:*)

DOUGLAS

Where are *my* papers?

ADELE

(*Avoiding him*) Calm, Stephen; it gets better. Here's the Carlinville Free-Democrat. It think's your improving.

DOUGLAS

Does it?

ADELE

(*Reads*) "Judge Douglas seems less bloated than in some of his past speeches."

DOUGLAS

I know that editor! He's a fanatic *abolitionist!* Come on, darling, where are my papers?

ADELE

Here are the good ones. I was saving them for dessert. (*Reads*) "Hundreds who had been applauding Lincoln all along, turned and applauded Douglas. At the end of the last debate, Lincoln was the worst used-up man in the United States."

DOUGLAS

That's more like it.

45

ADELE

The Philadelphia Press: "Poor Lincoln! He was writhing in
the powerful grasp of an intellectual giant."

DOUGLAS

(*Sits, puts his feet up on the table*) Go on, you're improving.

ADELE

Here's the best one of all. "Lincoln's Heart Fails Him! Lincoln's Legs Fail Him! Lincoln's Tongue Fails Him! Lincoln
Fails *All Over!*"

DOUGLAS

That's what I call clean, crisp reporting.

ADELE

Stephen, I wish there . . . (*Breaks off when she sees his feet
up*) Take your feet off the table.

DOUGLAS

Sorry . . .

ADELE

(*Taking up where she left off*) I wish there were some neu-
tral ground, where an *impartial* critic would say how it looks
to *him*. For perspective's sake, if nothing else. It's *silly* when
the Times reports a *thousand* torches in the torchlight parade
that met us in Freeport, whereas the Press and Tribune, because
it's for Lincoln, puts the number at only 74.

DOUGLAS

(*Laughing*) You can't let things like that bother you. Where
would we be if we tried to give the lie to every deliberate mis-
calculation and a slander?

ADELE

(*After a moment*) Yes . . . life would be nothing but a perpetual flea hunt, wouldn't it? (DOUGLAS *thinks this is a pretty shrewd comment, rises and embraces her appreciatively*)

DOUGLAS

"Perpetual flea hunt" . . . pretty good! (BLACKOUT) (*As they leave the stage, a spot comes up on our old friend the* REPUBLICAN COMMITTEEMAN. *He is excited about something contained on a piece of paper that he carries in his hand*)

REPUBLICAN COMMITTEEMAN

Good News! Good news for all Lincoln men! I'm informed a straw vote was taken on the excursion train from Oquawka yesterday with the results as follows:

> For Lincoln: 252 votes
> For Douglas: 116.

Out of sixty ladies in the train, 56 were for Lincoln—the great whole of the remainder for Douglas. So hurrah for Lincoln and the ladies! However, there is one item I'd like to take up which is an offense to the whole state of Illinois. (*Fishes in his pocket for a news clipping, as he goes on speaking*) I have received from a friend of mine in the nation's capital, a copy of the Norfolk Virginia Argus, in which it says: "The whole country is *disgusted* with the scene now being exhibited in the State of Illinois. The most malignant and reckless contest ever to disgrace the annals of American history is now being waged for the Senatorship. Ere long we expect the telegraph will tell us of a pugilistic encounter between the two candidates". I am going to reply to that slander. That's all I have to say. (*Off he goes. Now the principals return to the stage, as they did once before, in a half-light. When they are in position, the light comes up fast and* LINCOLN *resumes speaking:*)

47

There is a disadvantage under which I labor, and to which I ask your attention. It arises out of the relative positions of the two persons who stand before you as candidates. Senator Douglas is of world-wide renown. All the anxious politicians of his party have been looking upon him as certainly, at no distant day, to be President of the United States. They have seen in his round, jolly, fruitful face, post-offices, land-offices, marshalships, cabinet appointments, and foreign missions, bursting and sprouting out in wonderful exuberance, ready to be laid hold of by their greedy hands. And as they have been gazing upon this attractive picture so long, they cannot bring themselves to give up the charming hope; but with greedier anxiety they rush about him, sustain him, and give him marches, receptions, brass cannons, and triumphal entries. (ADELE *enters R, trying to be inconspicuous.* DOUGLAS *notices, puts his fingers to his lips.* LINCOLN, *too, notices her entry out of the corner of his eye; Adele sits in her chair*) In contrast to the Senator, the major portion of whose charm has just joined us—

(*Heartily*) At last, a true word, Mr. Lincoln—

(*Going on*) In contrast to the Senator, nobody expects *me* to be President. In my poor, lean, lank face, nobody has ever seen any cabbages sprouting. So you see, there *are* disadvantages under which we Republicans labor. (*Change of attack; soberly*) My friends—if we could first know where we are and whither we are tending, we could then better judge what to do and how to go about doing it. We are now far into the fifth year since a policy was initiated with the avowed object of putting an end to slavery agitation. Under the operation of that policy, that agitation has not only not *ceased*, but has constantly *increased*. In my opinion, it will not cease until a crisis shall have been reached and passed. Either the opponents of slavery will check the spread of it, or the advocates of it will push it until it becomes the law in all states, North or South. "A house divided against itself cannot stand." I believe this government cannot endure permanently half slave and half free. I do not expect the Union to be dissolved; I do not expect the house to fall; but I do expect it will cease to be divided. It will become all one thing or all the other. (*Sits*)

DOUGLAS

(*Rising and moving quickly to the attack*) "All one thing or all the other." . . . May I point out to Mr. Lincoln that his own Republican Party, in the northern part of the state, holds to an Abolition platform, but in the southern part it does not. I have seen Mr. Lincoln display varying shades of color, from jet black up in the northern counties, to a decent mulatto in the central part of the state, and almost white in the southern. (*Turns to* LINCOLN) So I now call down upon him the vengence of his own Scriptural quotation when I say his own *party* is a House Divided and cannot stand, and *ought* not to stand, for its attempt to mulct the American people out of their votes. In essence it comes down to this. My opponent is a two-faced man.

LINCOLN

Judge, I leave it to our audience. If I had another face, do you think that I would wear this one?

DOUGLAS

Whichever face you wear, Mr. Lincoln, you do it with distinction. —But unfortunately we must come to a matter of much graver concern. . . . Mr. Lincoln by his Scriptural quotation is inviting warfare between the North and South, to force our government to become all one thing or all the other. —Is sectional warfare to be waged between the Northern and Southern states merely because Mr. Lincoln says a house divided against itself cannot stand? . . . and pretends that this language of our Lord and Master is applicable to the American Union and the American Constitution? Surely Mr. Lincoln is a wiser man than those who framed our Government. Washington and the fathers of the revolution well understood that the laws and institutions which would suit the granite hills of New Hampshire would be totally unfit for the rice plantations of South Carolina, or the cranberry bogs of Indiana; they well understood that the great variety of interests in a Republic as large as this, required different regulations in each locality, and for that reason provided that the thirteen original states should remain supreme in regard to all that was local and internal, while the Federal Government should have certain powers which were general and national. I therefore conceive, Mr. Lincoln, that you have totally misapprehended the great principles upon which our Government rests. Uniformity in local affairs, I repeat, would be destructive of State sovereignty and personal freedom. Uniformity is the parent of *despotism* the world over!

LINCOLN

Judge Douglas thinks he has discovered a great political heresy. He says I'm in favor of making all the States uniform. I have said a hundred times that I believe the free states have no right to enter into the slave states and interfere with slavery where it exists . . . I have said that always. . . . Judge Douglas ha*s heard* me say it a hundred times.

DOUGLAS

Only in the southern part of the State, Mr. Lincoln.

LINCOLN

I believe each State has a right to do exactly as it pleases with all the concerns *within* that State, that interfere with the right of *no other* State. I do *not* believe in the right of Illinois to interfere with the cranberry laws of Indiana, the oyster laws of Virginia—or the liquor laws of Vermont, Judge Douglas. How then can Judge Douglas infer that, because I hope to see

slavery put in the course of ultimate extinction, I am in favor
of Illinois interfering with the oyster laws of Maine? —I suppose it's because he looks upon slavery as an exceedingly *little*
thing—this matter of keeping one-sixth of the population of
the nation in a state of tyranny unequalled in the world! He
looks upon it as being an *exceedingly* little thing—on a par
with whether a man shall pasture his land with cattle or plant
it with tobacco—as something having no *moral* question in it.
Well, it so happens there is a vast portion of the American
people who do *not* look upon that matter as a very little thing.
They look upon it as a *vast moral evil!* One of Judge Douglas'
chief arguments is that the authors of the Declaration of Independence did not intend to include Negroes, by the fact that
they did not at once actually place them on an equality with
the whites. (*To* DOUGLAS) Judge, this argument comes to just
nothing at all by the fact that they did not at once actually
place all *white* people on an equality with *one another.* They
did not mean to say all were equal in color, size, moral develop-
ment or social capacity. They defined, with tolerable distinct-
ness, in what respects they *did* consider all men created equal—
equal in "certain inalienable *rights*—among which are life,
LIBERTY, and the pursuit of happiness." This they said . . .
and this they meant. Let me pursue the Declaration for a moment. —The assertion that "all mean are created equal" was
of no practical use in effecting our separation from Great
Britain; it was placed in the Declaration, not for *that,* but for
future use. Its authors meant it to be, as, thank God, it is now
proving itself to be, a stumblingblock to all those who, in after-
times, might seek to turn a free people back into the hateful
paths of despotism. They knew the proneness of prosperity to
breed tyrants, and they meant that when such should reappear
in this fair land and commence their vocation, they should find
left for them at least *one* hard nut to crack! I have now ex-
pressed my view of the meaning of that part of the Declaration
of Independence which declares that all men are created equal.
—I should like to invite Judge Douglas to state *his* views on

the same subject. (*Turns, sees* DOUGLAS *whispering something to* ADELE, *his back to the audience and himself*) I see the Judge is not attending me just now.

DOUGLAS

(*Turning around*) I don't believe I've missed anything salient, Mr. Lincoln.

LINCOLN

Will you then state what you believe to be the meaning of the phrase, "All men are created equal"?

DOUGLAS

(*Caught by surprise; offbalance; brazening it out*) I believe the Declaration referred to the white race alone, and not to the African, when it declared all men to have been created equal . . . that it was speaking of British subjects on this continent being equal to British subjects born and residing in Great Britain—that they were entitled to the same rights.

LINCOLN

Thank you. —My good friends, think that over . . . and see what a mere wreck . . . a mangled ruin . . . it makes of our once glorious Declaration. Let me give you Judge Douglas's version of the text: "We hold these truths to be self-evident . . . that all British subjects who were on this continent 81 years ago, were created equal to all British subjects born and then residing in Great Britain." Why, according to the Judge, not only Negroes, but white people outside Great Britain and America were not spoken of in that instrument. The English, Irish, and Scotch, along with white Americans, were included, to be sure; but the French, Germans, and other white people of the world are all gone to pot along with the Judge's inferior races.

DOUGLAS

Demagoguery is not argument, Mr. Lincoln.

52

(*Ignoring the comment*) I had thought the Declaration promised something better than the condition of British subjects, but no, it only meant that we should be equal to them in their own oppressed and unequal condition. (*Stretches out his hands*) Now I appeal to all—are you really willing that the Declaration shall thus be frittered away?—thus left no more than an interesting memorial of the dead past?—no more than old wadding left to rot on the battlefield after the victory is won—shorn of its vitality, and left without even the *suggestion* of the individual rights of a man in it? This business of teaching that the Declaration of Independence has nothing to do with the Negro; that he ranks with the crocodile and the reptile; that man, with body and soul, is a matter of dollars and cents—these ideas, I say, are blowing out all the moral lights around us! (BLACKOUT. *A spot finds a* REPORTER, *who enters at downstage L. He is miffed about something, but preserves his dignity*)

REPORTER

I would like to address a few remarks to the Committee of Arrangements, if any of you are out there. Are you there?

A VOICE

(*From the audience*) Yes.

REPORTER

Well . . . as a reporter, and speaking for my colleagues of the working press, I want to say it's extremely difficult to do our job when our tables and chairs are jarred and overthrown by people on the platform. There are altogether too many idlers in the reporting area . . . and in every city, rabid partisans and drunks have come between us and the speakers. This is interfering with the accuracy of the reports. I hope you committee folk are aware that this is the first time newspaper correspondents have travelled with candidates or taken shorthand records of their speeches, and the experiment is being watched all over the country. So you can help us of the Press and your candidates too, by appointing officers strong enough to keep order on the platform and among the crowd. So . . . I'm sure it's little enough to ask, and it wouldn't inconvenience anybody, etc. . . . (*As he commences this final comment he moves down the steps to exit L, the pace of his speech and movement unrelenting, so that he is talking as he disappears*) *Now out of the darkness we see* ADELE. *She comes forward to address the audience. Under her speech—but not before—*LIGHT *rises on* LINCOLN *sitting in a leather chair, in a hotel lobby. As* ADELE *crosses to him, the* LIGHT *fades up until it is full by the time she reaches him.*

ADELE

(*To audience*) There was only one other time during the debates when I exchanged a few words with Mr. Lincoln. Stephen and I were staying at the Tremont House in Chicago and so was Mr. Lincoln. I met him in the lobby. Stephen had forgotten something, and had gone up to get it; Mr. Lincoln was sitting alone, in a big leather chair. (*Turns toward him*) He looked tired. I never saw a more thoughtful or dignified face. I never saw so sad a face.

LINCOLN

Good evening, Mrs. Douglas.

ADELE

Good evening, Mr. Lincoln. You look weary. Are you well?

LINCOLN

Oh, yes, thank you . . . but I *am* a little used up.

ADELE

So is the Senator. You certainly have had *at* each other.

LINCOLN

I'm afraid campaigning is not one of the gentler arts.

I had no illusions that you would be *tender* with each other,
but the *brickbats*—

Kind words about a man are usually saved up until after
he's dead . . . on the theory, I suppose, that they won't go to
his head then.

That *is* a little late for vanity.

Even post-mortem, of course, there's some question as to
how one will be treated when he gets where he's going. In the
cemetery up in New Salem, there's an epitaph on the grave of
an old Indian chief named Johnny Kangapod:

> "Here lies Johnny Kangapod—
> Be gentle to him, gracious God,
> As he would be if he were God,
> And You were Johnny Kangapod."

Now why can't you tell stories like that in the debates? I
mean when you both run out of arguments?

Do you think the Judge will ever let that happen?

Frankly, no.

Do you know the story of the backwoods housewife, who
lived in a messed-up log cabin? —One day a wandering
preacher came along and wanted to sell her a Bible. She answered sharply that she already *owned* a Bible. "Let's see it,"

said the preacher. So she started to look for it, but couldn't find it. She called in her children, and they joined in the hunt. At last, after turning the place upside down, one of the children held up in triumph a few torn and ragged pages of Holy Writ. The preacher tried to argue that this was no Bible and how could she pretend it was? But the lady stuck to her claims. "Of *course* it's a Bible," she said——"But I had no idea we were so nearly *out.*"

ADELE

(*Laughs*) Where *do* you get your stories, Mr. Lincoln? They are always so *apt*. It's uncanny!

LINCOLN

Maybe my ideas move in pairs, Mrs. Douglas, like the beasts entering Noah's Ark.

ADELE

I've heard it said that story-telling is characteristic of the country you were raised in.

LINCOLN

It's good enough country without stories, ma'am.

ADELE

I have no doubt.——Where Stephen was brought up, in Vermont, they're unusually tight-lipped.

LINCOLN

I believe that's one tradition he left behind him in New England. I say that very respectfully.

ADELE

I know you do. ——The last time we met, Mr. Lincoln, you mentioned your indifference to innuendo and insinuation. Since then I've read an attack on you that even I, in the camp of the enemy, know to be full of errors, if not outright lies. Do you mean to say you don't intend to write a letter setting the facts straight?

LINCOLN

I guess I'm not really mad enough. —Mrs. Douglas, I do the very best I know how. I mean to keep doing so. If the end brings me out all right, what's said against me won't amount to anything. If the end brings me out wrong, ten thousand angels swearing I was right would make no difference.

ADELE

But you seem to be a man of high principle. Is there no principle involved in this?

LINCOLN

Yes, but one picks carefully the principles he wants to stand up to defend. For example, a rich client came to my law office in Springfield one day, determined to sue a poor attorney for $2.50. I urged him to let the matter drop. I said, "You can make nothing out of him, and it will cost you a good deal more than the amount of the debt, for you to bring suit." But my client was determined to have his way. "Principle!" he said. "It's the *principle* of the thing!" So I finally took the case, and said my fee would be $10, which he paid me on the spot. As soon as he left the office, I hunted up the poor lawyer, told him about the suit, and handed him half of the $10. Together we went over to the squire's office, where he confessed judgment, and paid the $2.50 that he owed. That was the only way I could see to make things satisfactory—in principle—for my rich client as well as the poor debtor.

ADELE

(*Laughing*) A profitable deal all the way around.

LINCOLN

How are you bearing up under the debates, Mrs. Douglas?

ADELE

I'm not really. I find them frightening at times. I don't at all
like the way it's assumed in some quarters that the issue of war
and peace depends on you and my husband, as though you had
personally invented abolitionism, and he slavery. I have no
humor whatever when it comes to the subject of war. I think
it's the foulest abomination of mankind.

LINCOLN

I'm sure I feel just as you do about it.

ADELE

(*Sees* DOUGLAS *entering at R*) Well . . . the Judge will be
looking for me. One last question before I go, if I may: Was
the town of Lincoln in this state named after you?

LINCOLN

Well—all I can tell you is that *it* was named after *I* was.

ADELE

(*Smiling; as she starts off*) Good evening, Mr. Lincoln.

LINCOLN

Mrs. Douglas. . . . (*After* ADELE *has exited R,* LINCOLN *starts
slowly to cross toward his chair on the speaking platform. But
he is arrested by two musicians, a banjoist and flautist, who sit
on the pit step at downstage L, playing a haunting little melody.*
LINCOLN *stops, listens for a moment, then crosses up to his chair
and sits on it, continuing to listen until the music has ended
and the musicians exit. Then* ADELE *enters in the still half-light
and sits in her chair.* DOUGLAS, *entering last, reaches a position
on the forestage which indicates that he has been speaking for
some time as the* LIGHT *comes up quickly:*)

DOUGLAS

My fellow citizens, this is a young and growing nation. It
swarms as often as a hive of bees. In less than 15 years, if the

same progress continues, every foot of vacant land between
here and the Pacific Ocean will be occupied by the United
States. I tell you, increase, multiply, *expand*—that is the law
of this nation's existence! Indeed the time has now come, when
our interests would be advanced by the acquisition of the island
of Cuba. When we get Cuba, we must take it as we find it, leaving the people to decide the question of slavery for *themselves.*
When it becomes necessary to acquire any portion of Mexico
or Canada, we must take them as we find them, leaving the
people free to have slavery or not, as they choose.

LINCOLN

Then according to your view, new territory is to be acquired
as fast as it is needed?

DOUGLAS

Yes.

LINCOLN

Well, the indefinite part of *that* proposition is that we have
only you and your class of men to decide how fast it *is* needed.
(*To Audience*) The next thing, I suppose, will be a grab for
the territory of poor Mexico.

DOUGLAS

I believe I have the floor—

LINCOLN

When we get to Mexico, Judge, I don't know whether you'll
be in favor of the Mexican people that we get *with* it, settling
the slavery question for *themselves;* because you have a great
horror for mongrels, and I understand—from you—that the
people of Mexico are a *race* of mongrels. Wouldn't this bring
you into collision with your horror of inferior races?

DOUGLAS

(*Vehemently*) We have *seen* in Mexico the effects of this
mixture of superior and inferior races! —We have seen it in *all*

59

the Spanish-American States; and its results have been degeneration, demoralization, and degradation below the capacity for self-government! —I trust Mr. Lincoln will deem himself answered!

LINCOLN

Well, I don't, Judge.

DOUGLAS

(*Sardonically*) May I continue, Mr. Lincoln?

LINCOLN

I'm sorry, Judge, your time is up. (DOUGLAS *consults his watch, frowns, grunts "Oh, very well," and goes to his chair.* LINCOLN *rises*) Judge, did you ever hear about the farmer who said, "I ain't greedy about land—I just want all the land that's joined on to mine." Now I wonder, Judge, if you'd like to try answering another question. I want to read you something from the Missouri Republic. (*Fishes in his pocket and digs out a clipping, which he prepares to read by putting on specs*) I'm obliged to put on specs . . . my arms aren't long enough.

DOUGLAS

How touching.

LINCOLN

Now this is a report of a speech made by Judge Douglas recently, in which he describes me as being reluctant to face him on certain questions. I quote from the published account of his remarks: "I said frankly, to Lincoln, 'I intend to trot you down to Jonesboro.' The very notice that I was going to take him down there made him tremble in the knees so that he had to be carried from the platform. He laid up several days." Now that statement furnishes a subject for philosophical contemplations. I can explain it in no other way than by believing the Judge is crazy. If he was in his right mind, I cannot conceive how he would have risked disgusting the four or five

60

thousand of his own friends who knew that there was not a
word of truth in it.

DOUGLAS

(*Laughing*) *Didn't* they carry you off?

LINCOLN

There! There! That question illustrates the character of this
man Douglas *exactly*. He laughs now, and says, "Didn't they
carry you off?" But he said that I "*had* to be carried off:"
And he said it to convince the country that he had so com-
pletely broken me down by his speech that I had to be carried
away. Now he seeks to dodge it, and asks, "Didn't they carry
you off?" (*To* DOUGLAS) Yes, they did. But, Judge Douglas,
why didn't you tell the *truth* about it? You force me to admit
they carried me off *on their shoulders!—cheering!* Do I *look*
like being carried away trembling? Let the Judge go on; and
after he's done, I want you all, if I can't carry Judge Douglas
home to the hotel and put him to bed, to let me stay here and
rot!

DOUGLAS

(*Rises; to the audience, lightly*) Well, I did say there in
Joliet in a playful manner, that when I put certain questions
to Mr. Lincoln, he failed to answer, and that he trembled and
had to be carried off the stand, and required seven days to get
up his reply. (*To* LINCOLN) Do you deny that you didn't walk
off that stand?

LINCOLN

No.

DOUGLAS

Do you deny that a few persons took you off on their shoulders?

LINCOLN

No. . . .

61

Do you deny that they carried you through the streets?

No. . . .

(*To audience; in triumph*) I wish to say to you that whenever I *degrade* my friends and myself by allowing them to carry me on their backs through the public streets like some Asiatic potentate *when I am able to walk* on my own two feet, I am *willing* to be deemed crazy! (*Sits*)

Well, that's the Judge. . . . One more word, and I'm done. I hear people constantly argue that this Free State is not the right place to oppose slavery, because slavery *isn't* here; it must not be opposed in the Slave States, because it *is* there . . . it must not be opposed in *politics*, because that will make a fuss; it must not be opposed in the *pulpit*, because it is not religion. Then where *is* the place to oppose it? Judge Douglas has intimated that all this difficulty in regard to the Negro is the mere agitation of ambitious Northern politicians. Is that the truth? Doesn't it render even the churches asunder? Isn't it this same mighty, deep-seated power that operates on the minds of men, exciting and stirring them up in every avenue of society—in politics, in religion, in literature, in morals, in all the manifold relations of life? Is this the work of politicians? This power which for fifty years has shaken the Government and agitated the people, is it to be stilled and subdued by pretending that we ought not to *talk* about it? (*To* DOUGLAS) If you'll get everybody *else* to stop talking about it, I assure you *I* will quit before they do! These arguments that the inferior races are to be treated with as much allowance as they are capable of enjoying—what *are* these arguments? They are the arguments that kings have made for enslaving people in all ages of the world; they always bestrode the necks of the people, not that they *wanted* to do it, but because the people were better off for being ridden. This argument of the Judge is the same old serpent that says, "You work, and I eat; you toil, and I will enjoy the fruits of it." Turn it whatever way you will, whether it come from the mouth of a king as an excuse for enslaving the people of his country, or from the mouth of men of one race as a reason for enslaving the men of another race, it is all the same old serpent! If you take our old Declaration which declares that all men are equal, and say that it is not the truth, then let us take the statute book in which we find it and *tear it out!* (*Challengingly*) Who is so bold as to do it? If it is not *true*, let us tear it out! (*Waits for a response*) But if it *is* true, let's *stick* to it then: let's turn this Government back into the channel in which the framers of the Constitution originally placed it. Let us stand firmly by each other. Let's discard all quibbling about this man and the other man, this race and that race and the other race, being inferior. Let's discard all these things, and unite as one people throughout this land until we shall once more stand up declaring that all men *are* created equal! (HE *returns to his seat.* DOUGLAS *rises, takes the podium*)

DOUGLAS

In the remarks I make on this platform, I mean nothing personally disrespectful or unkind to Mr. Lincoln. There were many points of sympathy between us when we first got acquainted. We both struggled with poverty. I was a schoolteacher, and he was a grocery-keeper. I made as good a schoolteacher as I could, and when a cabinet-maker I made good bedsteads and tables, although my employer said I succeeded better with secretaries than with anything else. —Furniture, that is. I met Abe Lincoln in the State Legislature, and had sympathy with him, because of the up-hill struggle we both had in life. He was just as good at telling an anecdote then as he is now. He could beat any of the boys wrestling, or running a foot race; he could ruin more liquor than all of the boys of the town together; and the dignity with which he presided at a fist-fight excited the admiration and won the praise of everybody present. Whilst in Congress, however, Mr. Lincoln distinguished himself by his opposition to the Mexican War, taking the side of the common enemy against his own country; and when he returned home he found the indignation of the people followed him everywhere—and he was obliged to retire into private life, forgotten by his former friends. (LINCOLN *shoots up out of his chair and shouts with some heat:*)

LINCOLN

Just a minute! The Judge is at fault when he charges me with having opposed our soldiers in the Mexican War! He knows that whenever I was asked to indorse the origin and *justice* of the war, I refused to give such indorsement and voted against it; but whenever asked for money, or land grants, or anything to pay the soldiers in Mexico, during all that time, I gave the same vote that Judge Douglas did. You can think as you please as to whether that was consistent. Such is the truth, and the Judge has right to make all he can out of it! (*Sits*)

DOUGLAS

If Mr. Lincoln is a man of bad character, I leave you to find it out; if his course on the Mexican War was not in accordance with your notions of patriotism and fidelity to our own country as against a public enemy, I leave you to ascertain the fact. I have no assaults to make upon him, other than to trace his course. . . . (*With an air of summing up*) This is a contest of principle! Either the radical Abolition principles of Mr. Lincoln must be maintained, or the strong, constitutional, national Democratic principles with which I am identified.

LINCOLN

Yes, you have said that before. (*Jumping up*) Fellow citizens, if you were going to set about to devise the best instrument by which to change public sentiment in the free states to accept slavery, could you find an instrument so capable of doing it as Judge Douglas? He, by his vast personal influence and prestige, is in every possible way preparing the public mind for making the institution of slavery national and perpetual. THOSE are the principles by which he is identified. (*Sits*)

DOUGLAS

It has apparently not yet penetrated Mr. Lincoln's honorable brain that *his* principles are in every possible way preparing the public mind for *war* between the states!

LINCOLN

No!—

DOUGLAS

(*Forcefully*) Show me what is my duty in order to save the Union—and I will do it! —I am not for the dissolution of the Union under any circumstances! I will pursue no course of conduct that will give just cause for the dissolution of the Union! For the hope of the downtrodden and oppressed peoples of the world, the hope of the friends of freedom throughout the world, rests on the perpetuity of this Union. I am for peace forever between the States! (*The last big gun has been fired. The debate has ended in heat and passion, and some bitterness.* DOUGLAS *looks at his watch, comes down off the ramparts, speaks with deep sincerity, very much moved, to the audience*) And now my time, and the time of the debates, draws to a close. —I shall be satisfied whatever way you decide. If I was now to be consigned to private life, I would have nothing to complain of. I would even then, my dear fellow citizens, owe you a debt of gratitude which the balance of my life would not repay. (HE *returns to the platform.* LINCOLN *rises.* THEY *exchange a short nod, gather up their articles, and go off,* DOUGLAS R, LINCOLN L, *as the lights come down to* ADELE'S *narrative key.* SHE *comes forward*)

ADELE

That ended the debates, but not the rivalry. As you know, my husband was *not* consigned to private life. He was re-elected

65

and went back to Congress, while Mr. Lincoln went back to his law office. Stephen was jubilant, as was I. There was a great celebration in Springfield. Both candidates made statements, of a sort.

DOUGLAS

(*Coming on*) Let the voice of the people rule! (*Exits*)

LINCOLN

I feel like the boy who stubbed his toe . . . it hurt too bad to laugh, and he was too big to cry. But I'm glad I made the race. Though I now sink out of view and shall be forgotten, I hope I have made some marks which will tell for the cause of civil liberty long after *I'm* gone. (*Exits*)

ADELE

But the country had no intention of letting the rivalry rest there. Mr. Lincoln did not sink out of view, for the debates had made him a national figure, and two years later he was once more running against Stephen, this time for no less than the presidency of the United States. I confess to you that already I started thinking of the inaugural ball. There it was . . . the living prospect . . . to be the wife of a president of the United States! To be the first lady of a great land! How can I deny the brightness of that image . . . whenever my mind stole away, somewhat guiltily, to dwell upon it. (*There is the sound of a door closing*) Is that you, Stephen?

DOUGLAS

(*Entering*) Yes.

ADELE

I've been waiting for you. We mustn't be late for dinner. . . . (DOUGLAS *enters R carrying a newspaper.* ADELE *crosses to him, and her eye is caught by imperfections in his dress*) Stephen . . . your tie . . . it will never do for a president to slop about like a poet. . . . And how, Your Excellency, did you spot that waistcoat?

DOUGLAS

From natural causes.

ADELE

What natural causes?

DOUGLAS

Chicken gravy.

ADELE

Well, there will be federal spot cleaners in the White House.

DOUGLAS

I wouldn't worry too much about the White House if I were you, Adele.

ADELE

What is it, Stephen? What's wrong?

DOUGLAS

State elections. We've lost the governorship of Pennsylvania as well as a Senate seat in Indiana.

ADELE

What does that mean?

DOUGLAS

It's going to put the south in a wicked temper. And it can only widen the split in my party. How can the party stick together when the whole country's coming apart?

ADELE

And this plays into the hands of Mr. Lincoln?

DOUGLAS

I may as well tell you, Adele: Lincoln is bound to be our next President.

67

ADELE

(*Aghast*) How can you *say* that when only two States . . . and both of them local elections . . . ?

DOUGLAS

Two is a lot . . . and Lincoln is gaining strength in the North every day. But that isn't the ultimate danger. The *real* menace is not to my party or to me, but to the Union. It's come to a question of saving the *Union.*

ADELE

(*Incredulous*) Saving the Union?

DOUGLAS

I mean it. I'll never be President, but that's another matter. Something has to be done about the South, before the secession movement gathers too much force to be stopped.

ADELE

What can *you* do?

DOUGLAS

Go South. I've *got* to go *South,* and raise my voice as loud as I can, against the idea of secession! This country was meant to expand, to multiply, not divide! It will finish me off down there as far as any votes are concerned, but it's too late to worry about that.

ADELE

(*Protesting*) But you'll be practically campaigning for *Lincoln* if you go South!

DOUGLAS

That makes no difference. If I must lose the presidency because Lincoln and I see eye to eye on preserving the Union, then there are a lot worse causes and worse men that I could lose to.

68

ADELE

(*Passionately*) —But you just *can't* give up this way, Stephen! Great God in Heaven, how many men get a *chance* to run for the Presidency of the United States?

DOUGLAS

I'm not giving up any chances . . . they're gone anyway, with the party split the way it is. No—I've got to go South, that's all there is to it. . . . (*With a lingering hand on* ADELE, *he exits R.* ADELE, *disturbed, resumes speaking to the audience*)

ADELE

He went South. He spoke in a dozen cities. The Slave States didn't like his arguments against secession; he was threatened with physical violence all the time we traveled down there. In some places eggs were thrown at him . . . but he was not deterred for a moment. —And then came the election. Well, Stephen was the model of a good loser. I think I can say that with modesty and pride. On the very evening the Lincolns arrived in Washington an ailing Stephen called on the President at Willard's Hotel. . . . (DOUGLAS *enters from R,* LINCOLN *a moment later, from L. He greets* DOUGLAS *warmly, and offers him a chair*)

LINCOLN

Judge . . .

DOUGLAS

It's good to see you, Mr. President. (DOUGLAS *starts to sit, but holds up until* LINCOLN *precedes him.* LINCOLN *notices this, and motions for him to sit . . . a friendly waiving of formalities between them . . .*)

LINCOLN

No, no, sit down, sit down. . . . (*Concerned*) I've heard you're not well.

DOUGLAS

(*Dismissing it*) Oh, it's nothing. —Mr. President, we have said many harsh things to each other within the hearing of the whole country. But we have never, for a moment, disagreed in the conviction that the Union must not and shall not be destroyed. —I have come here tonight to assure you that I and my friends pledge ourselves with all our strength and energy to aid you. I am with you, Mr. President . . . and God bless you. (LINCOLN, *moved, looks at him silently.* HE *makes a move, a subtle indication that* HE *wants to reply . . . but perhaps an excess of emotion chokes him.* DOUGLAS *goes on*) I'm also concerned about the threats to do violence to you at the inauguration. Have the proper precautions been taken?

LINCOLN

If I were to worry about threats like that, I could never get on with this job.

DOUGLAS

Well, I want you to know that if any man attacks you, he attacks me too! I shall be there when you take the oath!

LINCOLN

(*After a moment*) Judge, when I first heard you called The Little Giant, I was satisfied that the name fitted—but you've never lived up to it more than you have just now. . . .

DOUGLAS

(*Moved*) Thank you.

LINCOLN

No, no—with all my heart I thank *you.* The people with us, and God helping us, all will yet be well.

DOUGLAS

I earnestly hope so. (*Rising*) Don't hesitate to call upon me if there's anything I can do.

LINCOLN

(*Slowly rising*) Well now, there may be. —As you know, there's trouble in our own state. The secessionists are busy again.

DOUGLAS

(*Shaking his head*) They never sleep, do they?

LINCOLN

We can take no chances of losing Illinois. As I remember now, you seem to have some influence back home. —Would you help me out by going there?

DOUGLAS

Of course I'd go. Whenever you say. I'd be honored to go.

LINCOLN

(*After a pause, in which* HE *studies* DOUGLAS' *face*) Thank you Stephen. Thank you. I'll never forget this.

DOUGLAS

Mr. President . . . (DOUGLAS *exits at stage R.* LINCOLN, *after a moment, slowly exits at L.* ADELE *enters from L and resumes narration*)

ADELE

On the day of the inaugural, on the platform itself, my husband stood just a little behind Mr. Lincoln, holding his hat. And at the Inaugural Ball that night, the President led the grand march, followed by Mrs. Lincoln hand-in-hand with Stephen. My husband and the first lady were partners in the quadrille. (*A little wistfully—this might have been herself*) To all of us it seemed that it must be the happiest night in her life. —Then, in spite of everything, or perhaps because of everything war came! The President did ask Stephen to go to Illinois, where there was growing anxiety. Tired and sick as he

71

was, Stephen went . . . and I went with him. (ADELE *retires to
the back of the platform, where* SHE *remains standing.* DOUGLAS
enters from L. HE *looks worn, haggard.* HE *is sick.* HE *has
trouble beginning his speech*)

DOUGLAS

(*Brokenly*) It is with a grief that I have never before ex-
perienced . . . that I contemplate this fearful struggle. —Bloody,
calamitous it will be. —But I believe in my conscience that it
is a duty we owe ourselves . . . and our children . . . and our
God . . . to protect this government, and our flag, from every
assailant . . . *BE HE WHO HE MAY!* (*Moves forward, as
though to be closer to his audience, as though to plead with
every last man*) Unite . . . unite as a band of brothers . . .
and rescue your Government . . . and its capital . . . and your
country . . . from the enemies who have been the author of our
calamity! (HE *finishes.* HE *is cold, clammy; sweat is on his
brow.* HE *is silent and still for a moment; then* HE *turns and
looks long, looks lovingly, silently at* ADELE. *With that,* HE
turns and very slowly walks off . . . a sick man, a dying man)
(ADELE *comes forward again, after which her husband leaves
. . . for what is the last time*)

ADELE

He saved Illinois for the Union. (SHE *pauses as though
affected emotionally, before* SHE *goes on*) Shortly after, Stephen
became very ill. It was in Chicago. He was worn out, exhausted.
And he had a strange fever. He became delirious . . . and yet
in his delirium his mind was taken with the nation's sickness
rather than his own. Once he cried out in his sleep: "Telegraph
to the President, and let the column move on!" At about 5
o'clock on the morning of June third, in his 48th year, he asked
that the blinds be thrown back and the window opened. He
seemed to revive for a moment, but then sank back on the
pillow and uttered the word "Death" three times. That was

the end. (*The lights dim.* LINCOLN *enters from the wing in a deep shadow, and speaks into the darkness:*)

LINCOLN

Drape the public buildings of the city in mourning, and the White House in deep black. Let all regimental colors be draped and in mourning also, in honor of this man who nobly discarded party for his country.

ADELE

Well . . . the war ground on. The blood of young Americans soaked into earth that should never have been contested. And it was not many seasons before the Capital was draped in black for the Commander-in-Chief himself. God knows that all of us who lived through those days, saw enough of struggle and anguish. At times the hatred and malice was thick about us, like a dense smoke. But when I was most discouraged, I remembered the principles that Stephen had stood for at the end; how he had worked for Union and for peace . . . and I remember also the words of his lifelong friend and opponent, back in the very year of the Debates, at a time when I gave them little heed . . . when it seemed to me that denying one man's rights couldn't possibly lead to trouble, so long as that man was inferior to others. . . . (LINCOLN *appears now in a dim, ghostly light, which has faded up unobtrusively during the fade down on* ADELE)

LINCOLN

What constitutes the bulwark of our liberty and independence? Not our frowning battlements, our army and navy . . . our defence is in the spirit which prizes liberty as the heritage of all men, in all lands everywhere. Destroy this spirit and you have planted the seeds of despotism at your doors. Familiarize yourself with the chains of bondage and you prepare your own limbs to wear them. Accustomed to trample on the rights of others, you have lost the genius of your own independence and become fit subjects for the first cunning tyrant who rises among you. Whether it is right or wrong to trample on the rights of others—that is the real issue . . . the issue that will continue in this country long after the poor tongues of Judge Douglas and myself shall be silent. (*The light fades, and the stage is in darkness*)

THE END

PROPERTY LIST

Preset: On Stage

On center platform:
  1 black table 30″ H, 20″ W, 36″ l:w/shelf
    on: 1 glass water pitcher w/4″ water
        2 8 oz. water glasses
  1 black bentwood chair UR platform (red seat)
  1 black wooden armchair L of table (red seat)
  1 black wooden armchair R of table (red seat)
Down Right Corner:
  1 wooden 4-leg table 30″ x 30″
  1 black bentwood chair above table

Off Left

 2 pocketwatches with chains
 1 folded white handkerchief (DOUGLAS)
 8 white addressed envelopes with letters
   (1 letter from Richard Merrick from script)
 1 letter from Lincoln to Douglas (no envelope)
 1 rolled sheet 8½ x 11 paper (DOUGLAS)
 1 long-necked whiskey bottle
   in: 6″ strong cold tea
 1 quill pen (with ball point pen inserted)
 1 black pen holder
12 sheets white bond paper
 6 newspaper clippings on 4 x 6 cards with text from script
   written out
 1 red bandana (LINCOLN)
 1 news clipping on 5 x 7 card (written out) for DOUGLAS
 1 needle threaded with black thread
 1 train coach seat
 1 large carpetbag
 1 round felt-covered table
 1 armchair with leather seat

1 green leather cushioned armchair
1 green leather seat stool
1 practical shotgun with blank shell loaded
1 small silver hip flask
1 folded white handerchief
1 folding fan
1 blue hat (DOUGLAS)
1 small carpetbag
1 folded newspaper

PERSONAL

LINCOLN

1 pr. eyeglasses
1 black pencil
1 stovepipe hat
   in: small notepaper
1 3 x 5 white card
2 notes written from text
   (Supreme Court decision)
   (copy of article from Missouri
      Republic)
1 red bandana

COMMITTEEMAN

1 pr. eyeglasses
1 newspaper

PROPERTY MOVES

ACT I

At end of ADELE's narration, "To hear their champions speak"
   COMMITTEEMAN   Strike DR table off R2
   REPORTER   Strike DR chair off R2

At CUE LIGHT OP (Start of First Debate):
   SHOTGUN BLAST UR

At CUE LIGHT end of First Debate:
   BAND ENTER FROM PIT and as cymbal player exit L:
   REPORTER set bentwood chair DR, and hold for ADELE to sit

At end of COMMITTEEMAN's speech, he strikes chair off R2

After Lady Democrat's entrance from pit:
   TOWNSMAN & COMMITTEEMAN set Train Seat DL
                              carpetbag R of seat

During interval:
> PROPS Strike train seat off L
> Set table DL
>> on: pen holder
>> pen
>> 8 sheets white paper
>> pocketwatch
>> whiskey bottle

Act II

At start of Committeeman's speech:
> TOWNSMAN   Strike table and handprops off L
> REPORTER   Strike chair off L

At cue, "This is interfering with the accuracy of the reports."
during REPORTER speech:
> COMMITTEEMAN   Set stool and armchair DR
> TOWNSMAN   Strike railing from platform off L

At start of BANJO-FLUTE VIGNETTE on forestage:
> COMMITTEEMAN   Strike stool off R
> TOWNSMAN   Strike chair off R

WARDROBE LIST

LINCOLN

1 black frock coat	1 black stovepipe hat
1 black vest	2 plain front white shirts
1 pr. black trousers	4 black bow ties

1 pr. black boots

DOUGLAS

1 double-breasted blue frock coat	1 blue top hat
	3 pleated white shirts
1 grey vest	2 bow ties
1 pr. grey trousers	1 pr. black shoes

1 hair fall

COMMITTEEMAN

1 grey frock coat	1 grey soft hat
1 vest	2 white shirts
1 pr. tweed trousers	1 black bow tie
1 pr. black shoes	2 wing collars

REPORTER

1 blue frock coat	2 hats
1 vest	2 shorts
1 pr. trousers	1 bow tie

TOWNSMAN

1 dark green frock coat	2 white shirts
1 vest	1 tie
1 pr. herringbone trousers	1 pr. black shoes

1 soft black hat

LADY DEMOCRAT

1 plaid dress	1 pr. shoes
1 straw bonnet	1 pr. white gloves
1 petticoat	1 pr. gold earrings

MUSICIANS

5 uniforms	2 vests
(black trousers, red coats)	2 pr. trousers
5 band uniform caps	4 buff shirts
5 pr. black shoes	2 soft light hats

ADELE

1 grey dress	1 pr. white Pantaloons
1 blue dress	1 pr. black shoes
1 red velvet dress	5 stoles: white, lilac, black,
black & red velvet head-dresses	blue lace, garnet stripe
1 flower half-dress	3 pr. earrings: blue, garnet,
1 silver purse	gold
2 beaded bags	2 velvet neck jewels
2 grey hats	1 grey cape
1 black hat	3 slips
1 lilac hat	1 hoop skirt

3 pr. stockings

COSTUME PLOT ADELE DOUGLAS

ACT I

Opening	Grey dress without hat
1st Inning	Blue dress / with hat with plume, white organdy scarf
Fanning Scene	Blue dress / no hat, change scarf or no scarf
2nd Inning	Blue dress / small shawl, violet hat

78

ACT II

Opening Scene	Red dress / gay apron
3rd Inning	Red dress / blue dolman, hat
Lobby	Red dress / remove dolman, remove hat, add stole and flower comb
Final Inning	Red dress / hat, cape or another jacket (reversible) (perhaps—change into black skirt during Willard Hotel scene)

MUSIC CUES

1. Overture: As stage lites fade to black and ADELE enters into the follow
2. End Scene I: Fife and Drum Band, then brass band over
3. End First Debate: Band enters playing a march and Exit as completing march
4. End Interval: Banjo player on forestage, plays 1 minute
5. End Lobby Scene (II-17): Banjo and Flautist play forestage
6. Under Lincoln's Speech (II-30) Trumpet and Tympany
7. End Act II: Trumpet and Tympany Crescendo

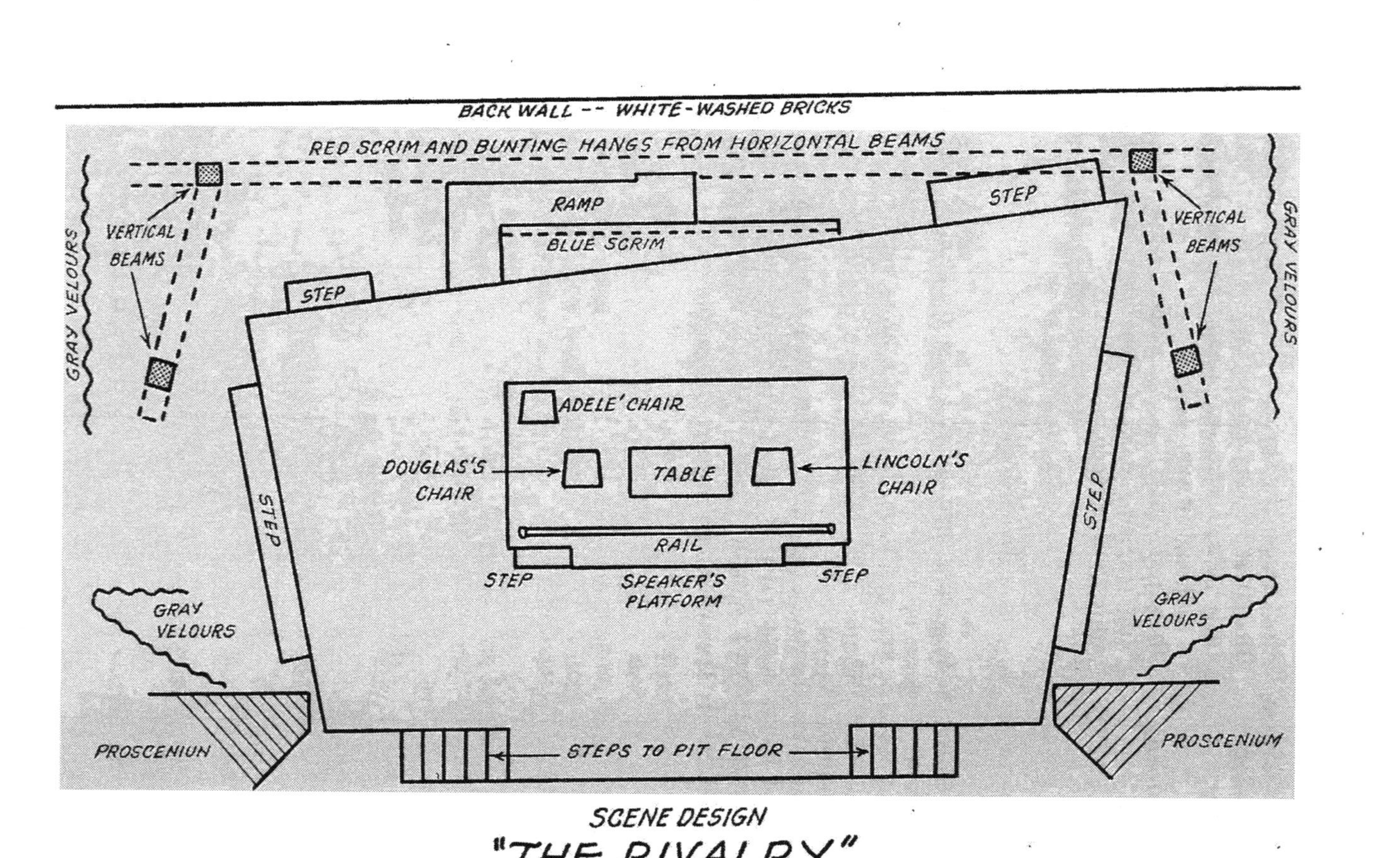

SCENE DESIGN
"THE RIVALRY"

Recent Plays

THE TEAHOUSE OF THE AUGUST MOON
THE GREAT SEBASTIANS
THE SOLID GOLD CADILLAC
A VIEW FROM THE BRIDGE
THE LARK
THE SEVEN YEAR ITCH
BAD SEED
SEVEN NUNS AT LAS VEGAS
THE TENDER TRAP
A ROOMFUL OF ROSES
BUS STOP
ANNIVERSARY WALTZ
SOMEONE WAITING
RECLINING FIGURE
KING OF HEARTS
SABRINA FAIR

Dramatists Play Service, Inc.

14 East 38th Street   New York 16, N. Y.

Printed in the USA
CPSIA information can be obtained
at www.ICGtesting.com
CBHW070802190524
8716CB00069B/1140